an a-z of

baby names

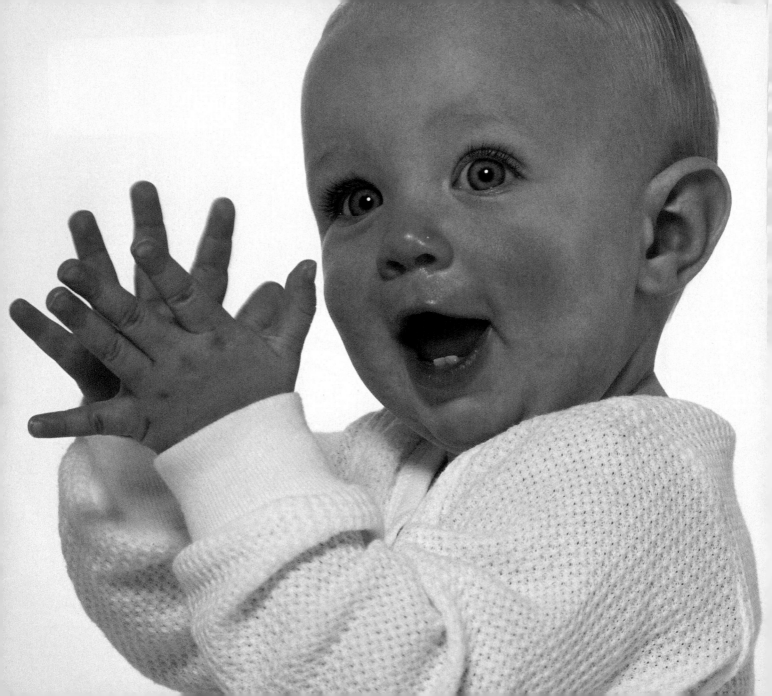

an a-z of
baby names

igloobooks

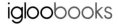

Published in 2014
by Igloo Books Ltd
Cottage Farm
Sywell
NN6 0BJ
www.igloobooks.com

LEO002 0314
2 4 6 8 10 9 7 5 3
ISBN 978-1-84561-769-1

Cover photograph courtesy of Image Source
Contents photographs courtesy of Punchstock

Designed by seagulls

Printed and manufactured in China

Introduction

If choosing a name for your baby seems a daunting task, it may be made easier by working through a few practical considerations to help you narrow your field of choice – which is colossal, as this book shows.

It's worth thinking about how a name will suit your baby's last name (or family name). Names that rhyme with a last name seldom sound as melodious as those that don't rhyme. In the same way, if a last name begins with a vowel, it's probably best to steer away from first names that end in a vowel; the risk is that the names may be run together and lose their individuality.

The way your baby's name will be written, more particularly any word that the initials inadvertently spell, needs bearing in mind as well.

Names that form a pun with your last name might amuse you, but having to live with the combination year in year out for your child's entire life is a very different matter. So names like Brandon Hyde, Amber Light, or Poppy Flowers are also best avoided as well.

A lot of parents like to name their babies after family members or close friends, both of which will provide an immediate source of familiar names to set you thinking. Family traditions and religious preferences may also play an important part in your selection.

The meaning of a name might help you settle on one from a shortlist of favorites, so the origins and meanings of names form an important part of this book.

If you decide you would prefer your child not to be one of several sharing the same name at school or among their friends, you might be drawn to a less familiar name – something unique that will make them stand out from the crowd. However, a name that is so unusual that no one has ever heard it or knows how to pronounce or spell it can be an embarrassment. Many parents find a successful combination in fitting an unfamiliar first name with a well known last name and vice versa.

Ultimately, the name you decide to give your baby is down to you and this book aims to make choosing it enjoyable and interesting no matter how long it takes.

Aaron
Origin/meaning: Hebrew 'high mountain' or Egyptian (no known meaning).
Aaron was the brother of Moses and first High Priest of Israel. Used as a first name after the 16th-century Reformation.
Variations: Aron (Eng), Aharon (Heb), Haroun (Ar).

Abbas
Origin/meaning: Arabic 'stern'.
Abbas, 566–652, was an uncle of Mohammed and became one of the Prophet's most ardent supporters. He was the founder of the Abbasides, Khalifs of Baghdad, 750–946.
Variation: Abasi (Swahili).

Abdul
Origin/meaning: Arabic 'servant of God'.
This is one of the commonest Muslim names, and is found in slightly varying forms in many countries.
Variations and abbreviations: Abdu (worshipper of God) (Swahili), Abdala (Swahili), Abdullah.

Abel
Origin/meaning: Hebrew 'breath' or 'son'.
Abel was the second son of Adam and Eve, killed by his brother Cain.
Variations and abbreviations: Abe, Abell, Able, Nab.

Abelard
Origin/meaning: Old German 'noble resolution' from 'adal' – 'noble', 'hard' – 'resolute'.
The French and best-known version of the name.
Variations and abbreviations: Adalard (Eng), Adalhard (Old Ger), Alard.

Abhay (pron. Ahbpóy)
Origin/meaning: Sanskrit/Gujerati, 'fearless'.

Abraham
Origin/meaning: Hebrew 'father of a multitude' from the Hebrew word 'abba' – 'father'.
The name of the Patriarch of Israel whose name was changed by God from Abram to Abraham (Genesis ch.17). This was one of the names brought into use in the 13th century in England. Now more popular in the US than Britain because of President Abraham Lincoln. The contraction Bram is popular in the Netherlands and US.

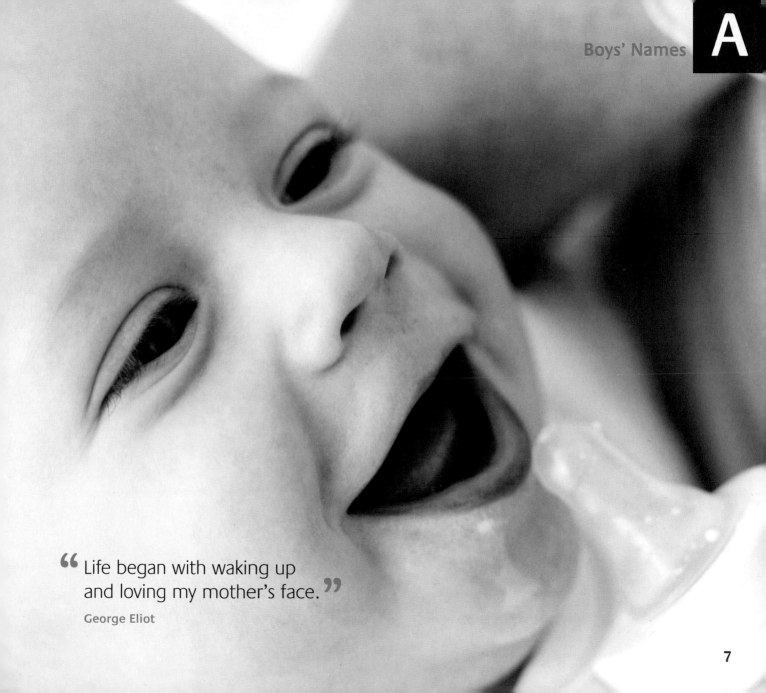

"Life began with waking up
and loving my mother's face."
George Eliot

Boys' Names

Variations and abbreviations: Abe, Abey, Abie, Abrahamo (It), Abrahán (Sp), Abram, Abramo, Avram, Avrom, Bram, Ibrahim (Ar), Ham.

Absolom
Origin/meaning: Hebrew 'father of peace'.
The name of King David's son by Maacah (Samuel I + II). Popular in the 12th and 13th centuries.
Variations and abbreviations: Absolon (Fr), Axel (Ger/Scand).

Achilles
Origin/meaning: Greek. May mean 'tight-lipped' or be connected with the River Achellos.
Still common in Greece and where there are large Greek communities.
Variation: Achille (Fr).

Adam
Origin/meaning: Hebrew 'red (earth)'.
In the Book of Genesis Adam, the first man, was fashioned from the earth and is presumed to have taken his name from its color. Adam became popular in Britain in the 13th century especially in the North. Many last names derive from it, e.g. Adams, Adamson, Atkins, MacAdam.
Variations and abbreviations: Ad, Adamh (Ir), Adamnan, Adamo (It), Adan (Sp), Adda (Wel), Addan, Adao (Port), Ade, Edom (Scot).

Ade
Origin/meaning: Yoruba 'royal'.

Adolph
Origin/meaning: Old German 'noble wolf'. The English version of Adolphus.
Variations: Adolf (Ger), Adolphe (Fr).

Adrian
Origin/meaning: Latin 'from Adria' (the port which gave its name to the Adriatic Sea).
One of the best-known holders of this name is the Roman Emperor Hadrianus, who built Hadrian's Wall in the North of England to keep out the Scots. It did not become well known until the 12th century when Nicholas Breakespear became the first (and only) English Pope, taking the name Adrian IV.
Variations and abbreviations: Adriaen, Adrien (Fr), Arrien, Arne.

Ahmed
Origin/meaning: Arabic 'praiseworthy'.
This popular name is found in all Muslim countries in the same form. It was the name of three Turkish Sultans in the 17th and early 18th centuries.

Aidan
Origin/meaning: Old Irish 'little fire' or 'little fiery one'.
The name of an influential 7th-century Irish saint who converted the North of England to Christianity.
Variations: Adan, Eden.

Akbar
Origin/meaning: Sanskrit 'the great'.
This was the epithet applied to the great Mogul Emperor Jelal-ed-din-Mohammed, 1542–1605. In a few years he extended his Empire to the whole of India north of the Vindhya Mountains. He was a wise and humane ruler who practiced religious tolerance.

Akiiki (pron. Akee-éekee)
Origin/meaning: Muneyankole 'friend'.

Alan
Origin/meaning: 'handsome'.
A name originally introduced into England at the time of the Norman Conquest from Brittany, the Celtic area of France. It was originally found in its French form, Alain.
Variations and abbreviations: Ailean (Scot), Ailin (Ir), Al, Alain (Fr), Aland, Alano (It/Sp), Alein, Allan, Allayne, Allen, Alleyn.

Alastair
Origin/meaning: Ancient Greek 'defender of men'.
A Scottish form of Alexander q.v.
Variations and abbreviations: Al, Alasdair, Alistair, Alister, Allister.

Alban
Origin/meaning: Latin 'white', 'fair'.
This name has appeared consistently since at least AD 287 when St Alban was martyred at the Roman town of Verulamium, later named St Albans in his honor.
Variations: Albany, Alben, Albin (Ger), Albion, Alva (Sp), Aubin (Fr).

Albert
Origin/meaning: Old German 'noble bright' from 'adal' – 'noble', 'berhta' – 'bright'.
Its real popularity in the present form is almost entirely due to Queen Victoria's marriage in 1840 to the German Prince Albert.
Variations and abbreviations: Adalbert, Ailbert (Scan), Al, Alberto (It/Sp), Albrecht (Ger), Aubert (Fr), Bert, Bertie, Halbert.

Aldous
Origin/meaning: Old German 'old'.
One of the many 13th-century additions to the number of English first names. Usually found both as a first name or a last name on the East Coast of England.
Variations and abbreviations: Aldis, Aldo, Aldus.

Boys' Names

Aldred
Origin/meaning: Old English 'old counsel'.
An Anglo-Saxon name still found occasionally after the Norman Conquest.

Alec
Origin/meaning: Ancient Greek 'defender of men'.
One of the many variations of Alexander q.v.
Variations and abbreviations: Alek, Aleck, Alic, Alick.

Alexander
Origin/meaning: Ancient Greek 'defender of men'.
The name of the famous Greek conqueror Alexander of Macedon, 356–323 BC, it has been popular ever since. It is particularly popular in Scotland which has had several kings of that name. In Scotland it frequently takes the form Alastair.
Variations and abbreviations: Al, Alasdair (Scot), Alastair (Scot), Alaster, Alec, Alejandry (Sp), Alek, Aleksandr (Russ), Alessandro (It), Alex, Alexan, Alexandre (Fr), Alexio (Port), Alexis, Alic, Alick, Alisander, Alistair (Scot), Alister, Allister, Sacha, Sander, Sandro (It), Sandy, Sasha, Saunder.

Alexis
Origin/meaning: Ancient Greek 'helper' or 'defender'.
Popular in Russia and Greece, Alexis has recently become more popular in English-speaking countries. Also a short form of Alexander q.v. Sometimes found as a short form of the girl's name Alexandra q.v.

Alfie
Origin/meaning: Old English 'elf-wise counselor' hence 'good counselor'.
A short form of Alfred, Alfie is now a very popular first name in its own right, probably due to the lead character from the 1966 Michael Caine film 'Alfie' that was remade with Jude Law in 2004.

Alfred
Origin/meaning: Old English 'elf counselor', 'good counselor'.
This was the name of one of the Saxon Kings of England, Alfred the Great, 849–901.
Variations and abbreviations: Al, Alf, Alfie, Alfredo (It/Sp), Alfy, Alured, Avery, Fred, Freddie, Freddy.

Algernon
Origin/meaning: Norman French 'bearded', 'with whiskers'.
This name began as a nickname some 900 years ago at a time when most men were clean-shaven.
Abbreviations: Algie, Algy.

Ali

Origin/meaning: Arabic 'exalted'.
Ali, d.661, was the cousin of the Prophet Mohammed, and the first convert to Mohammedanism. He married the Prophet's youngest daughter, Fatima q.v. He was fearless in his devotion to the Prophet and became Khalif, but was later assassinated.

Aloysius (pron. Allowíshus)

Origin/meaning: Old German 'glorious battle'.
It developed as the Latin, written form of the old Provençal name Aloys, meaning son of Loys (Louis). A 16th-century St Aloysius, one of the early Jesuits, popularized the name in Catholic Europe.
Variations and abbreviations: Alois (Ger), Aloisio (It), Aloisius, Aloys. See also Louis.

Alphonso

Origin/meaning: Old German 'adal-funs' – 'noble and ready'.
Now a comparatively rare name except in Spain where it was introduced in the 8th century.
Variations and abbreviations: Affonso (Port), Alfons (Ger), Alfonso (Sp/It/Scand), Alonzo, Alphonse (Fr), Alphonsus (Lat/Ir), Fons, Fonsie, Fonz, Fonzie.

Alvin

Origin/meaning: Old German 'noble friend'.
A form of the Old English name Aylwin q.v. which is more usually found in America.
Variations: Aloin (Fr), Aluin, Alvan, Alwin (Ger).

Amadeus

Origin/meaning: Latin 'beloved of God'.
Uncommon in English-speaking countries.
Variations and abbreviations: Amadeo (Sp/It), Amadis, Amado, Amando, Amédé (Fr).

Ambrose

Origin/meaning: Greek 'divine', 'immortal'.
The Greek gods fed on Ambrosia which ensured their immortality. St Ambrose, a 4th-century saint, made the name popular.
Variations and abbreviations: Ambie, Ambrogio (It), Ambros (Ir/Ger), Ambrosi, Ambrosio (Sp), Ambrosius (Ger/Scand), Amby, Emrys (Wel).

Amos

Origin/meaning: Hebrew 'burden' or 'bearer of burdens'.
A minor prophet of the Old Testament.

Boys' Names

André
Origin/meaning: Greek 'manly'.
A French form of Andrew q.v.

Andrew
Origin/meaning: Greek 'manly'.
St Andrew, one of Jesus's Apostles, was an immensely popular saint who was patron saint of Scotland and Russia. In England the name came into use after the Conquest. The old Scottish short form Dandy, became synonymous with a man who is over-interested in his appearance.
Variations and abbreviations: Anders (Scand), Andie, André (Fr), Andrea (It), Andreas (Ger/Dut), Andres (Sp), Andy, Drew.

Aneurin (pron. An-eye-rin)
Origin/meaning: Latin 'honorable'.
A common name in Wales. There was a 7th-century Welsh bard of that name whose poem 'Y Gododdin' describes a famous Welsh attack on the English at Catterick.
Variations and abbreviations: Aneirin, Neirin, Nye.

Angus
Origin/meaning: Old Gaelic 'one choice'.
A common name in Scotland. It is found in early legends and was the name for a 9th-century saint. It has an Irish Gaelic equivalent – Aonghus, pronounced the same way.
Variations and abbreviations: Aonghus (Ir), Aeneas, Gus.

Anselm
Origin/meaning: Old German 'helmet of God'.
A Lombard name brought to England after the Norman Conquest. The name of a 12th-century saint, who was Archbishop of Canterbury.
Variations and abbreviations: Anseaume (Fr), Anselmo (Ir), Elmo.

Antony
Origin/meaning: Latin – Antonius. The name of one of the great families of Rome. Meaning uncertain but is sometimes given as 'beyond price'.
The best known early holder of this name was Mark Antony, the famous Roman soldier and lover of Cleopatra. Two saints – St Antony the Great, 4th century, and St Antony of Padua, 13th century – helped to establish the popularity of the name. The alternative spelling, Anthony, appeared at the end of the 16th century. In the US, the name is sometimes pronounced with a soft 'th' sound instead of a hard 't'.
Variations and abbreviations: Anthony, Antoine (Fr), Anton (Ger/Scand), Antoni, Antonio (It/Sp/Port), Antonius, Tony.

> "The sweetest flowers in all the world – a baby's hands."
>
> Swinburne

A

Boys' Names

Archibald
Origin/meaning: Old German 'genuinely bold'.
This name has become unfashionable except in parts of Scotland.
Variations and abbreviations: Archaimbaud (Fr), Archambault (Fr), Archibaldo (Sp), Archibold, Archie, Archy.

Archie
Origin/meaning: Old German 'genuinely brave'.
This short version of Archibald has now become a far more popular first name than the original form.
Variation and abbreviation: Archy.

Arnold
Origin/meaning: Old German 'eagle-power'.
Brought to England by the Normans at the time of the Conquest, Arnold was very popular for several centuries, often in the French form Arnaud. Many last names derived from it, e.g. Arnott, Arnett, Arnell.
Variations and abbreviations: Arnoldo (Sp), Arnaud (Fr), Arni, Arnie, Arnoldo (It), Arny.

Arran
Origin/meaning: As in the Isle of Arran. Occasionally used as a male name.

Arthur
Origin/meaning: Old Welsh 'bear' or Old Irish 'stone' or Latin 'Artorius' (one of the patrician Roman families).
Early versions of the name were 'Arter' and 'Artar'. The 'h' appears around the 16th century. It did not become popular until the 19th century, with the revival of interest in medieval history and the legend of King Arthur and his Knights of the Round Table, coupled with the popularity of the victor of Waterloo, Arthur Wellesley, Duke of Wellington.
Variations and abbreviations: Art, Artair (Scot), Arte, Arttois (Fr), Artie, Artur (Ir), Arturo (Sp/It), Artus (Fr), Arty.

Asher
Origin/meaning: Hebrew 'happy'.
Asher was one of the sons of Jacob by Zilpah, the maid of his wife Leah. He was the founder of one of the tribes of Israel. The name is found both as a last name and first name among Jewish people.

Ashley
Origin/meaning: Old English 'ash tree wood' or 'clearing'.
A widespread English last name which became popular during the 19th century when many last names were adopted as first names.
Variations and abbreviations: Ash, Ashlin.

Ashok (pron. Assówk)

Origin/meaning: Sanskrit 'tree'.
Ashok, 269–233 BC, was one of the most famous Indian Emperors. His symbol is incorporated into the modern Indian flag. During his reign Buddhism became widespread. He encouraged builders to use stone so their buildings would last.
Variations: Ashoka, Asoka.

Ashton

Origin/meaning: Old English 'ash tree settlement'.
This last name is now used as a first name, most commonly in the US.
Variation and abbreviation: Ash.

Athol

Origin/meaning: Old Scots 'new Ireland'.
The name of an area of Scotland found both as a last name and first name.
Variation: Atholl.

Auberon (pron. Oberon)

Origin/meaning: Old German 'little elf-ruler'.
Diminutive English form of the German Alberich, from its French version Auberi. It was not unusual in Medieval England. Shakespeare used the alternative spelling Oberon as the appropriate name for the King of the Fairies in 'A Midsummer Night's Dream'.
Variations and abbreviations: Oberon, Bron.

Aubrey

Origin/meaning: Old German 'elf-ruler'.
The English form of the German Alberich comes from its French version Auberi, as does Auberon q.v. Common in Medieval England.
Variations: Alberich (Ger), Alberik, Albery, Avery.

August

Origin/meaning: Latin 'venerable', 'majestic'.
A version of the old Roman name Augustus that is now found as a name in its own right. It is originally a German form of the name.

Augustus

Origin/meaning: Latin 'venerable', 'majestic'. A title given to Roman emperors.
Brought to England by the Hanoverians in the 18th century, it was popular for about a century and was the second name of Queen Victoria's husband Albert.
Variations and abbreviations: Agosto (It), Aguistin (Ir), Agustin, Augie, August (Ger), Auguste (Fr), Augustin, Augustine, Augusto (Sp), Austen, Austin, Augy, Gus.

A

Boys' Names

Avinash (pron. Aveenass)
Origin/meaning: Sanskrit 'indestructible'.
This is a Hindu name.

Axel
Origin/meaning: Hebrew 'father of peace'.
The Scandinavian and German form of Absolom q.v.

Azikiwe (pron. Azeekiwi)
Origin/meaning: Ibo 'vigorous'.
This is a name found in Nigeria.
Abbreviation: Zik.

Aziz
Origin/meaning: Arabic 'precious'.
This name is popular among Muslims.
Variation: Azizi (Swahili).

B

Babar
Origin/meaning: Sanskrit 'tiger'.
This Muslim name was first used as an epithet to Zahir-ud-Din-Mohammed, 1493–1530, the first of the Muslim Mogul Emperors of India. The character in French children's literature, Babar the elephant, is named after him.
Variation: Babur.

Badhur
Origin/meaning: Arabic 'born at the full moon'.
A popular Muslim name.
Variations: Badar, Badr, Badru (Swahili).

Bailey
Origin/meaning: various origins, English 'bailiff' or 'town dweller'.
This old last name is now found as a first name especially in the US and is also used for girls.

Barry

Origin/meaning: Old Irish 'spear'.
An exclusively Irish name until the 19th century when Irish emigrants spread it further afield.
Variation: Barrie.

Bartholomew

Origin/meaning: Hebrew 'son of Tolmai', 'son of a farmer'.
This is the patronymic (father's name) of the Apostle Nathanael, and the name by which he is best known. St Bartholomew was immensely popular in Medieval England.
Variations and abbreviations: Bart, Bartelmy, Barthel (Ger), Barthelemy (Fr), Bartholomé (Fr), Bartolome (Sp), Bartholomeus (Scand/Dut), Bartholomeo (It), Bat.

Baruch

Origin/meaning: Hebrew 'blessed'.
The name of the companion of the prophet Jeremiah. Popular in the 17th century like many other Biblical names.

Basil

Origin/meaning: Greek 'kingly'.
A popular name in the Eastern Christian Church because of St Basil the Great, 330–379. The name was probably brought to Western Europe by the Crusaders.
Variations and abbreviations: Baz, Basile (Fr), Basilio (It/Port/Sp), Basilius (Dut/Ger/Scand), Vasilis, Vassily (Slav/Russ).

Benedict

Origin/meaning: Latin 'blessed'.
A common name in England after the Norman Conquest. An old form is Benedick, used by Shakespeare in 'Much Ado About Nothing'. Its original popularity was largely due to the honor in which St Benedict, 480–547, the founder of the Benedictine Order, was held.
Variations and abbreviations: Ben, Bendix, Bendt (Dan), Benedetto (It), Benedicht (Swiss), Benedick, Benedicto (Sp), Benedikt (Ger/Scand), Benet, Bengt (Swed), Bennet, Bennett, Benito (It/Sp), Bennie, Benny, Benoit (Fr).

Benicio

Origin/meaning: Spanish 'benevolent person'.
The popularity of this Spanish name in the English-speaking world is mainly due to the Hollywood actor Benicio Del Toro.

Benet

Origin/meaning: Latin 'blessed'.
An English short form of Benedict q.v., more widespread in the Middle Ages than the original.
Variations and abbreviations: Ben, Benett, Bennet, Bennett.

B

Boys' Names

Benjamin

Origin/meaning: Hebrew 'son of my right hand'.

In the Book of Genesis, ch.35, Rachel, Jacob's second wife, died giving birth to a son whom she called Ben-oni 'son of my sorrow'. He was then renamed by his father Benjamin 'son of the south' or 'son of my right hand'. The name Benjamin has come to be synonymous with a much loved youngest son.

Variations and abbreviations: Ben, Beniamino (It), Benji, Benjie, Bennie, Benny.

Bernard

Origin/meaning: Old German 'bear-hard', Old English 'noble and strong'.

A name popular in England for several centuries after the Norman Conquest. Often used to honor St Bernard of Clairvaux, 1091–1153, founder of the Cistercian Order of Monks.

Variations and abbreviations: Barnard, Barnet, Barney, Bearnard (Ir/Scot), Berend (Ger/Dan), Bern, Bernardo (It/Sp), Bernd (Ger), Berne, Bernhard (Ger), Bernt (Swed), Bernie, Berny, Burnard, Burnhard.

Bertram

Origin/meaning: Old German 'brilliant raven'.

One of many names brought to England at the time of the Norman Conquest. The raven was the device of Odin, Norse god of war.

Variations and abbreviations: Bart, Bartram, Beltrame (It), Beltrán (Sp), Bert, Bertie, Bertran, Bertrand (Fr), Bertrando (It), Berty.

Bevis

Origin/meaning: Old French, meaning uncertain. May be 'boy' or 'young calf'.

A name brought over by the Normans in 1066. Never widely popular.

Bharat (pron. B'rat)

Origin/meaning: Sanskrit 'the sustainer'.

This is one of the names of the Hindu god of fire Agni. He became a famous king and gave to the country the name (pron. Bhaar't), which many Indians still use today instead of India.

Bill

Origin/meaning: Old German 'will helmet' i.e. 'helmet of resolution'.

A popular short form of William q.v. sometimes given as an independent name.

Björn

Origin/meaning: Old German 'bear'.

The Scandinavian form of Bern, one of the short forms of Bernard q.v. Now widely known in English-speaking countries because of the former Swedish tennis champion Björn Borg.

Variation: Beorn (Med Eng).

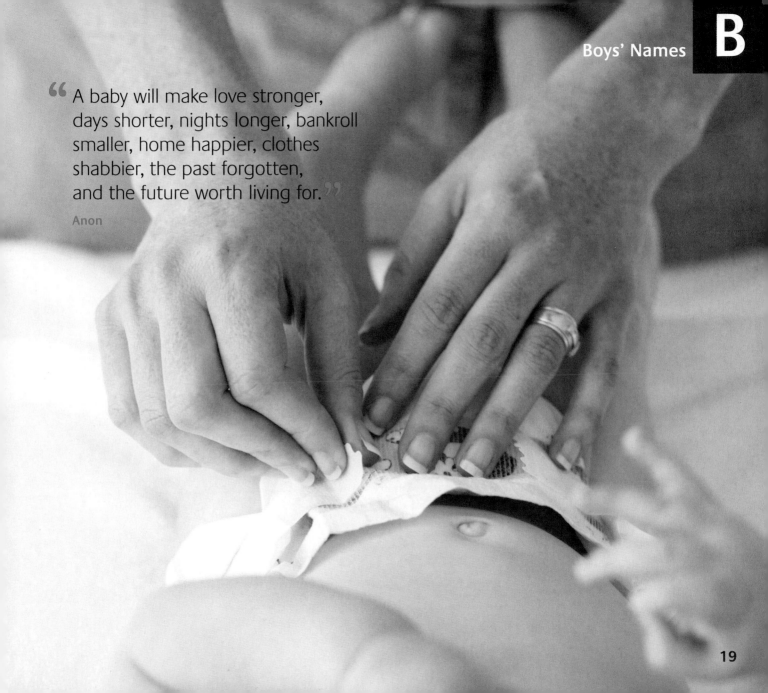

"A baby will make love stronger, days shorter, nights longer, bankroll smaller, home happier, clothes shabbier, the past forgotten, and the future worth living for."

Anon

B

Boys' Names

Blake
Origin/meaning: Old English 'pale' or 'black'.
An English family name not uncommon as a first name in the US perhaps because of its short 'masculine' sound.

Blase
Origin/meaning: Latin 'stammerer' or possibly French 'from Blois'.
This name seems to go back to the martyr St Blaise, d.316. He was the patron saint of wool carders. The popularity of his name in Medieval England may well be due to the great importance of the wool industry at that time.
Variations and abbreviations: Biagio (It), Blaise (Fr), Blas (Sp), Blasien (Ger), Blasius (Ger/Latin), Blayze, Blaze.

Boris
Origin/meaning: Old Slav 'fighter', 'warrior'.
A popular Russian name, short for Borislav.

Brad
Origin/meaning: a short form of many family names e.g. Bradford, Bradley. Used, in the US especially, as a given name.

Bradley
Origin/meaning: Old English 'broad clearing'.
An English place-name used as a family name and used in the US as a given name. Also popular in Australia.
Abbreviation: Brad.

Brandon
Origin/meaning: Old English 'gorse hill'.
This old place name became a last name and then finally a first name. It is especially popular in the US.
Variations and abbreviation: Brand, Branden.

Brayden
Origin/meaning: Old English 'wide valley'.
This name is popular in the US.
Variation: Braydon.

Brendan
Origin/meaning: Old Irish 'dweller by the flame' or 'dweller by the beacon'.
An Irish name, correctly pronounced without the d. St Brendan was a 6th-century Irish saint and according to legend the first discoverer of America.
Variations: Brandan, Brandon, Brendin, Brenainn (Ir Gaelic), Brennan.

Brett

Origin/meaning: Old English/Old French 'Breton'.
Particularly popular in the US.

Brian

Origin/meaning: Celtic (probably Old Irish) from the word 'strength' or 'hill'.
A Celtic name introduced to England from Brittany at the time of the Conquest.
Variations: Briano (It), Briant, Brien, Brion, Bryan, Bryant, Bryon.

Broderick

Origin/meaning: Old Welsh 'son of Roderick'.
A family name used, particularly in the US, as a first name.

Brook

Origin/meaning: Old English 'brook'.
A common last name used as a first name, particularly in the US.
Variation: Brooks.

Brooklyn

Origin/meaning: Place name, borough of New York City.
England soccer star David Beckham and his wife Victoria named their first child in honour of where he was conceived – Brooklyn in New York. As a result Brooklyn has emerged as a fashionable given name.

Bruce

Origin/meaning: a place name, Braöse/Brieuse (modern) in Normandy.
This was brought over to Britain as a last name – de Braöse or de Bruce – at the time of the Norman Conquest. The family was very influential and widespread. One member, Robert the Bruce, 1274–1329, became King of Scotland and defeated the English at Bannockburn.
Variation: Brucie.

Bruno

Origin/meaning: Old German/Old English 'brown'.
Used in the Middle Ages to honor St Bruno, 1033–1101, the founder of the Carthusian Order of Monks.

Bryn

Origin/meaning: Old Welsh 'hill'.
Rare outside Wales.

Boys' Names

Bud

Origin/meaning: US familiar term for 'brother'.
Usually a nickname but sometimes used as a given name.
Variations and abbreviations: Budd, Buddie, Buddy.

Byron

Origin/meaning: Old English 'at the cowsheds'.
A place name from the North of England from which the name of Lord Byron, the English Romantic poet, derived.
Variations: Byram, Byrom.

C

Cadell

Origin/meaning: Old Welsh/Old Scots 'spirit of battle'.
Found as a first name in Wales and a family name in Scotland.
Variation: Cadel.

Cai (pron. Kay)

Origin/meaning: from the Roman family name Gaius which is derived from the verb 'to rejoice'. This Roman name is still used today in Wales. It is more familiar in England as Kay q.v. who was one of the Knights of the Round Table.
Variations and abbreviations: see Kay.

Calum

Origin/meaning: Latin/Scottish 'dove'.
Calum is a form of the old Latin name Columba. Its recent popularity may be linked to Calum Best, celebrity son of former soccer star George Best.
Variations and abbreviation: Callum, Cally.

Calvin

Origin/meaning: Latin 'bald'.
John Calvin, 1509–1564, the religious reformer, was a hero figure among Puritans, especially those who went to America.
By the 18th century his last name was being used as a first name.
Variations and abbreviations: Cal, Calv, Vin, Vinny.

Cameron
Origin/meaning: Old Scots 'crooked nose'.
A Scottish clan-name used as a first name.
Abbreviation: Cam.

Carl
Origin/meaning: Old German 'man'.
This is a German form of Charles q.v. now used as a separate name in its own right.
Variations: Karl, Carlo (It).

Carlos
Origin/meaning: Old German 'man'.
The Spanish and Portuguese form of Charles that has become prevalent in the US.
Variation and abbreviation: Carlo.

Carson
Origin/meaning: origin unknown.
A name from Scotland and Northern Ireland that was first used in the 13th century as a last name.

Cary
Origin/meaning: Old English place name from the Somerset area.
As a first name, it was popularized by film star Cary Grant.

Casimir
Origin/meaning: Polish 'command of peace'.
The English and French version of a Polish name.
Variations: Casimiro (It), Kasimir (Ger), Kazimierz (Pol), Kazmer.

Caspar
Origin/meaning: uncertain, possibly Persian.
Sometimes, because of the legend of the three wise men, said to mean 'treasurer'.
Variations and abbreviations: Casper, Cass, Cassie, Kaspar (Ger), Kasper. See also Jasper.

Cassius
Origin/meaning: Latin 'vain'.
Cassius is the name of one of the men who plotted against Julius Caesar in Shakespeare's play.
Variations and abbreviations: Cass, Cassie, Cassy.

Boys' Names

Cecil
Origin/meaning: Latin – Caecilius – one of the patrician families of Rome. Probably from the Latin word for 'blind'.
One of many aristocratic family names (in this case of the Marquis of Salisbury) used as a masculine first name from the
19th century.

Cedric
Origin/meaning: uncertain. Possibly Old Welsh 'war chief'.
Used by Sir Walter Scott for one of his characters, Cedric the Saxon in 'Ivanhoe', 1820. Its use for the hero of Frances Hodgson
Burnett's popular book 'Little Lord Fauntleroy', 1886, reinforced its popularity.

Ceredig
Origin/meaning: a character from Welsh legend. Ceredig was the son of Cunedda. He gave his name to the area Ceredigion.

Chandler
Origin/meaning: Old French/English 'candle maker'.
An old family name that came from an occupation, it has been given a new lease of life thanks to the character Chandler Bing,
played by Matthew Perry, in the TV comedy series 'Friends'.

Charles
Origin/meaning: Old German 'man'.
This was the name of the Holy Roman Emperor Charlemagne – 742–814. The German form of the name was Karl, Latinized in
documents as Carolus. In France it developed into Charles, the name of many French kings.
Variations and abbreviations: Carl, Carlo (It), Carlos (Sp), Carrol, Carroll, Cary, Caryl, Charley, Charlie, Chick, Chuck, Karel, Karl,
Karol (Pol).

Chase
Background: Norman 'huntsman'.
Far more common as a first name in the US than in Britain.

Chester
Origin/meaning: Latin/Old English 'fortified camp'.
A place name which became a common family name now found, mainly in the US, as a given name.
Abbreviation: Chet.

Chris
Origin/meaning: Latin 'Christian' or 'Christ bearer'.
A short form of Christian, Christopher or Christine q.v., sometimes used as an independent name.
Variations: Cris, Kris.

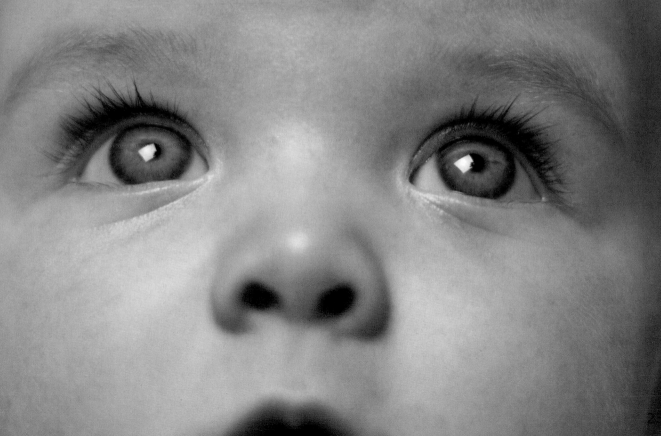

> " Sweet babe, in thy face
> Soft desires I can trace, Secret joys and
> secret smiles, Little pretty infant wiles. "
>
> **William Blake, Infant Joy**

Boys' Names

Christian
Origin/meaning: Latin 'Christian'.
Especially popular in Denmark which has had several Kings of that name.
Variations and abbreviations: Chrétian (Fr), Chris, Chrissy, Christiano (It/Sp), Kristian (Sp).

Christopher
Origin/meaning: Greek 'Christ bearer'.
This is one of the earliest Christian names. It was applied to a legendary saint who was supposed to have carried the infant Christ across a river. St Christopher thus became the patron saint of all travelers.
Variations and abbreviations: Chris, Chrissie, Chrissy, Christie, Christoffer (Dan), Christoforo (It), Christoph, Christophe (Fr), Christophonis (Ger), Christy, Chrystal, Cris, Cristóbal (Sp), Cristoforo (It), Cristoval (Sp), Kester, Kit, Kristoff (Scand).

Chuck
Origin/meaning: 'man'.
US familiar form of Charles q.v.

Clarence
Origin/meaning: Latin 'bright', 'famous'.
An English Royal title. Lionel, son of Edward III, was given the title Duke of Clarence in 1362, because his wife was heiress of the Clare family.

Clark
Origin/meaning: Old French 'scholar'.
A common English last name which has become a first name, particularly in the US.
Variations: Clarke, Clerk.

Claud
Origin/meaning: Latin 'lame'. The name of a patrician Roman family.
Introduced to England from France in the 16th century.
Variations: Claude (Fr), Claudian, Claudianus (Ger), Claudio (It/Sp), Claudius (Ger/Dut), Klaudius (Ger). See also Antony, Cecil.

Clem
Origin/meaning: Latin 'gentle', 'merciful'.
A short form of Clement sometimes found as an independent name, particularly in the US.

Cliff
Origin/meaning: Old English 'ford at a cliff'.
Short form of Clifford, the family name of Baron Clifford of Chudleigh, and occasionally of other last names. Frequently used as an independent name.

Clinton
Origin/meaning: Old English 'from the headland farm'.
An English last name used as a given name.
Abbreviation: Clint.

Clive
Origin/meaning: Old English 'at the cliff'.
The last name of Robert Clive, 1725–1774, the Englishman largely responsible for annexing India for the East India Company. His last name became popular as a first name.

Cody
Origin/meaning: Old English 'cushion'.
Has become a widely-used name in the US, probably in honor of the Wild West hero William Frederick Cody, better known as Buffalo Bill.
Variation: Codie.

Colan
Origin/meaning: Old Cornish 'dove'.
Colan is the Old Cornish version of the Latin Columba.

Colin
Origin/meaning: Greek/Old French 'victory of the people' or Old Scots 'young man'.
The name came to England from France in the Middle Ages as a diminutive of Nicholas. The Scottish name is sometimes considered to be yet another variation on the name Columba, 'dove'.
Variations and abbreviations: Cailean (Scot), Col, Colán (Ir), Cole, Collin.

Colum
Origin/meaning: Latin 'dove'.
This Irish name is one of several Celtic forms of Columba. Their popularity resulted from the great prestige of St Columba among people in Celtic areas.
Variations and abbreviations: Col, Cole, Colm. See also Colan, Colin, Malcolm.

Conan (pron. Cóe-nan; Irish, Connáwn)
Origin/meaning: Old Irish 'high', 'mighty' or 'intelligent'.
A widely found Celtic name.
Variations and abbreviations: Con, Conal, Conn, Conny, Kynan.

Boys' Names

Connor
Origin/meaning: Old Irish 'high desire'.
An extremely popular Irish name.
Variations and abbreviations: Con, Connaire (Ir), Conn (Ir), Conor.

Conrad
Origin/meaning: Old German 'bold counselor'.
Variations and abbreviations: Con, Conn, Connie, Conrade (Fr), Corrado (It), Corradino (It), Cort (Dan), Curt, Koenraad (Dut), Konrad (Ger/Scand), Kurt.

Conway
Origin/meaning: Old Welsh 'holy water' or Old Irish 'hound of the plain'.
The name possibly originated from the place-name Conway in Wales. Generally a last name, it is now a regularly used first name.
Variations and abbreviations: Con, Conn, Connie, Conny.

Cormac
Origin/meaning: Old Irish 'charioteer'.
An Irish last name and first name, it features in many of the pagan Irish myths and legends.
Variations and abbreviations: Cormack, Cormick, Mac.

Cornelius
Origin/meaning: the Cornelius family, one of the great families of Ancient Rome.
The name may come from the Latin 'horn' which implied kingship. There were several saints of the name. One of these was martyred and his remains eventually taken to the Low Countries. The cult surrounding him made the name popular in the Netherlands and also among descendants of the early Dutch settlers in the United States, such as the Vanderbilt family.
Variations and abbreviations: Con, Conn, Connie, Connor, Conny, Cornel, Cornelis (It/Sp), Cornell, Corny, Cory.

Cosmo
Origin/meaning: Greek 'order', 'harmony', 'the universe'.
SS Cosmas and Damian were, according to legend, twin brothers, who practiced as doctors without charging money. The Medici family, Dukes of Florence, adopted the form Cosimo as a family name which popularized it further.
Variations and abbreviations: Cos, Cosimo (It/Sp), Cosmé (Fr).

Courtenay
Origin/meaning: either Old French 'short nose' or de Courtenay, an aristocratic family from Courtenay in France.
The family name of the West Country Earls of Devon. It was particularly successful in the US.
Variations and abbreviations: Court, Courtnay, Curt.

Craig
Origin/meaning: Old Scots/Old Welsh 'crag'.
One of the most common Scots last names, based on several place names and popular as a given name.

Crispian/Crispin
Origin/meaning: Latin 'curled'.
Crispinianus and Crispinus were two shoemakers who were both martyred, probably in the 3rd century. They became the patron saints of shoemakers.

Cruz
Origin/meaning: Spanish 'cross'.
England soccer star David Beckham and wife Victoria named their third son Cruz, a Spanish name, while the baby's father was playing for Real Madrid.

Curt
Origin/meaning: a short form of names like Conrad, Courtney, Curtis. Used as a given name, particularly in the US.
Variation: Kurt.

Cyril
Origin/meaning: Greek 'lordly'.
St Cyril, 827–869, with his brother, took Christianity to the Slavs. They were aided by their knowledge of Slav languages. They devised a script to write these languages down, known as Cyrillic, which is still used today for the Russian language.
Variations: Cirille (Fr), Cirillo (It), Cirilo (Sp), Cyrill (Ger), Cyrillus (Dut), Kyrill (Ger), Kyrillus (Ger).

Cyrus
Origin/meaning: Persian/Greek 'throne'.
Cyrus the Great, 560–629, first Persian king and a powerful ruler, surrounded by fable and legend. The name is popular in the US.
Variations and abbreviations: Ciro (It/Sp), Cirus, Cy, Russ.

D

Dai
Origin/meaning: Hebrew 'darling', 'friend'.
A popular Welsh short form of David q.v. from Dewi and Dafydd.

Boys' Names

Dale
Origin/meaning: Old English 'from the valley'.
An English last name used as a first name, usually for boys.
Variations and abbreviations: Dael, Dal.

Damian
Origin/meaning: Greek 'tamer'.
Damian and Cosmas were two early Christian martyrs who probably died in Syria.
Variations and abbreviations: Dami, Damiano (It), Damien (Fr), Damyan.

Daniel
Origin/meaning: Hebrew 'God has judged' or Old Irish 'dark-haired'.
Daniel was a Hebrew prophet who was delivered from the lions' den where he had been thrown by the Persian king Darius. The 17th-century Puritan liking for Biblical names gave it an extra boost.
Variations and abbreviations: Dan, Daniele (It), Danilo (Slav), Danni, Dannie, Danny, Deiniol (Wel).

Darby
Origin/meaning: Old Irish 'free from envy' or English 'from Derby'.
The use of Darby in the phrase 'Darby and Joan', meaning an inseparable old married couple, dates back to 1735.
Variation: Derby.

Darcy
Origin/meaning: Old French 'from Arcy', Old Irish 'dark man'.
This is a name that came to England as a last name with William the Conqueror. It became an Irish first name after a branch of the family settled there in the late Middle Ages.
Variations: D'Arcy, Darsey, Darsy.

Darren
Origin/meaning: uncertain. Sometimes given as Old Irish 'little one' or Greek 'from Doris'.
This appeared in the 1960s and 70s and is a last name used as a first name. An American television series of the early 1960s in which the main character's name was Darren helped to spread it, reinforced by the concurrent popularity of US singer Bobby Darin.
Variations: Daren, Daron, Darrin.

Daryl
Origin/meaning: Old English 'little dear', 'darling'.
A very old name still used occasionally today.
Variations and abbreviations: Darrel, Darrell, Darryl, Daryll.

"A new baby is like the beginning of all things –
wonder, hope, a dream of possibilities."
Eda J. Le Shan

D

Boys' Names

Daud
Origin/meaning: Arabic 'beloved'.
A widespread Muslim name similar to David q.v.
Variations: Daudi (E Africa), Dauvud.

David
Origin/meaning: Hebrew 'darling' or 'friend'.
King David, who slew Goliath and is reputed to have written the Psalms, is one of the outstanding characters in the Bible. The 6th-century Welsh saint Dewi (David) founded many monasteries, chief among them being at Mynyw, now known as St David's. The Scots had their own St David, 1084–1153, who was also their king, David I. The name was therefore well established in both Scotland and Wales before it was introduced into England at the time of the Norman Conquest.
Variations and abbreviations: Dai (Wel), Dafydd (Wel), Dave, Davidde, Davide (Fr/It/Sp), Davie, Davin, Davy, Deio (Wel), Dewey (Wel).

Dean
Origin/meaning: 'from the valley'.
An English last name used as a first name.
Variations: Deane, Dene, Dino.

Declan
Origin/meaning: origin unknown.
This old Irish name has recently become extremely popular though it is often shortened to Dec. Declan is the real first name of singer Elvis Costello.
Abbreviation: Dec.

Denis
Origin/meaning: Latin/Greek 'follower of Dionysos'.
The Greek name Dionysius was a common one because of the popularity of the god of fertility and wine. A St Dionysius, who took Christianity to what is now France, was beheaded at Montmartre (the hill of the martyr) in Paris in 258. He was adopted as the patron saint of France and known as St Denys.
Variations and abbreviations: Den, Denness, Dennet, Denney, Dennis, Denny, Denys (Fr), Dion, Dionisio (It/Sp), Dionys (Ger), Dionysius (Ger).

Denzil
Origin/meaning: uncertain, possibly Latin/Greek 'follower of Dionysos'.
A Cornish last name used as a first name since the 17th century.
Variation: Denzell.

Derek

Origin/meaning: Old German 'ruler of the people'.
This name is from the Old German Theodoric. In the late Middle Ages trade with Holland introduced the Dutch forms Diederick and Dirk, from which the 20th-century spelling Derek evolved.
Variations and abbreviations: Dedrik, Deric, Deryk, Derrick, Diederich (Ger), Diederick (Dut), Dietrich (Ger), Dirk.

Dermot

Origin/meaning: Old Irish 'free from envy'.
This is an Anglicized form of the Irish Diarmaid. Diarmaid in Irish legend ran off with Grainne, Queen of Tara. Her husband forced Diarmaid to fight with a wild boar which killed him.
Variations: Darby, Derby, Dermott, Diarmid, Diarmit.

Desmond

Origin/meaning: Old Irish 'from South Munster'.
This is an Irish last name which came into general use as a first name in the 19th century.
Abbreviation: Des.

Dexter

Origin/meaning: Old English 'dyer'. Sometimes given as Latin 'right-handed', 'dexterous'.
An English last name sometimes used as a first name.

Dhruva (pron. Dhroov)

Origin/meaning: this is the Hindu name for the pole star.
Dhruva is a character from Indian mythology. Rejected by his father, King Uttanpada, he went into the forest and gradually achieved spiritual perfection through meditation. On his death the gods transformed him into Dhruva-Loka, the pole star.

Digby

Origin/meaning: Old English 'settlement by a ditch'.
An English place name which became a last name and has been occasionally used as a given name.

Diggory

Origin/meaning: French 'lost', 'strayed'.
An old-fashioned name, possibly Cornish, rare nowadays.

Dillon

Origin/meaning: Old Irish 'faithful' or Old German 'destroyer'.
An Irish last name sometimes used as a first name.

Boys' Names

Dinesh
Origin/meaning: Hindi/Gujerati 'helper of the poor'.

Dion
Origin/meaning: Latin/Greek 'follower of Dionysus'.
A form of Denis q.v.

Dirk
Origin/meaning: Old German 'ruler of the people'.
A Dutch form of Theodoric. It has been found in England since the late Middle Ages when England was engaged in the wool trade with Holland.
Variations: Dierk (Ger), Derk.

Dominic
Origin/meaning: Latin 'of the Lord'.
A name either intended to dedicate a child to God or to indicate he was born on a Sunday, the Lord's day. It gained wider use in the Middle Ages when it was given to honor St Dominic, 1170–1221, founder of the Dominican Order of Friars.
Variations and abbreviations: Dom, Domenic, Domenico (It), Domingo (Sp), Dominick, Dominique (Fr), Nick, Nickie, Nicky.

Donald
Origin/meaning: Old Scots 'world ruler'.
The name of six Scottish kings, Donald is, not surprisingly, one of the commonest Scottish names. The short form Don/Donen can have the independent meaning 'dark', and is found in several last names which are sometimes used as given names, such as Donovan, Donnelly and Donahue.
Variations and abbreviations: Don, Donal (Ir), Donalt, Donn, Donnie, Donny.

Donovan
Origin/meaning: Old Irish 'dark warrior', 'brown warrior'.
Abbreviation: Don.

Dorian
Origin/meaning: Greek 'from Doris' (one of the famous areas of classical Greece).
This is the male version of Doris q.v. Made famous by Oscar Wilde's novel 'The Picture of Dorian Gray', 1891.
See also Dylan.

Dougal (pron. Doogal)
Origin/meaning: Old Irish 'dark stranger'.
Used by the Irish as a term for Scandinavian invaders it became a general Celtic term used by Irish, Scots and Bretons for strangers.
Variations and abbreviations: Doug, Doyle (Ir), Dug, Dugald, Duggie.

Douglas

Origin/meaning: Old Irish/Scots 'from the dark water'.

This is a common descriptive place or river name. The famous Scottish clan name Douglas developed as a first name within the family, when it was given as a name to both male and female children.

Variations and abbreviations: Doug, Dougie, Douglass, Dougy, Dug, Duggie.

Drew

Origin/meaning: Old German 'bearer' or Old French 'vigorous'.

This is the Medieval English form of the name Drogo, by way of the French form Dru. Drogo lost its popularity after the 17th century but Drew survives, in the US particularly.

Variations: Drogo, Dru.

Duane (pron. Dwayne)

Origin/meaning: Old Irish 'small and dark'.

A 'new' first name popular in the US in the 1950s and 60s perhaps because of the guitarist Duane Eddy and also its similarity to another 60s favourite, Wayne.

Variation: Dwayne.

Dudley

Origin/meaning: Old English 'Dudda's clearing'.

Dudda was a Saxon nobleman, and Dudley is a town in the English West Midlands. The Dudley family was one of the fastest rising families in Tudor England, eventually being granted the Earldom of Leicester. The family name was not used as a first name until the 19th century.

Abbreviation: Dud.

Duncan

Origin/meaning: Old Irish 'brown headed'.

Like many names of Irish origin this was quickly adopted by Scotland whose language was so similar. There were two Scottish kings of that name, the first of whom is the Duncan, 1034–1040, murdered by Macbeth and well known from Shakespeare's play.

Abbreviations: Dun, Dunc, Dunk.

Dwight

Origin/meaning: uncertain, possibly Old French 'from the Isle of Wight' or Old Flemish De Witt, 'from Witt'.

A last name, it became a first name in the 19th century particularly in North America.

Dylan (pron. Dúllan)

Origin/meaning: Old Welsh 'dark' often given as 'from the sea'.

A character from Welsh legend whose father was the God of the Sea.

Variations and abbreviations: Dill, Dillan, Dillon, Dullan.

E

Eamon
Origin/meaning: Old English 'prosperous protector'.
The Irish form of Edmund q.v.
Variation: Eamonn.

Earl
Origin/meaning: Old English 'nobleman' or 'warrior'.
This is an English last name which probably indicates an ancestor was in the service of an earl. Since the 19th century this family name has been used in the US as a first name.
Variations: Earle, Erle.

Ebenezer
Origin/meaning: Hebrew 'stone of help'.
This is a Biblical place name referred to in the first Book of Samuel. It was popular among the 17th-century Puritans. It declined in popularity, partly because of the unattractive character Ebenezer Scrooge in 'A Christmas Carol' by Charles Dickens.
Variations and abbreviations: Benezer, Eben.

Ebner
Origin/meaning: Hebrew 'father of light'.

Eden
Origin/meaning: Hebrew 'delight' or Old English 'rich'.
The second meaning refers to Eden when used as a form of Ede and Edith q.v. during the Middle Ages.

Edgar
Origin/meaning: Old English 'rich spear'.
Edgar (Eadgar) was one of the names used by the royal house of Wessex. Its royal usage together with hopes of a Saxon revival, may account for the survival of the name for several centuries after the Norman Conquest.
Variations and abbreviations: Eadgar, Ed, Edgard (Fr).

Edmund
Origin/meaning: Old English 'rich guardian'.
As in Edward, Edgar and Edith the first syllable of this name indicates it was used by the royal house of Wessex before the

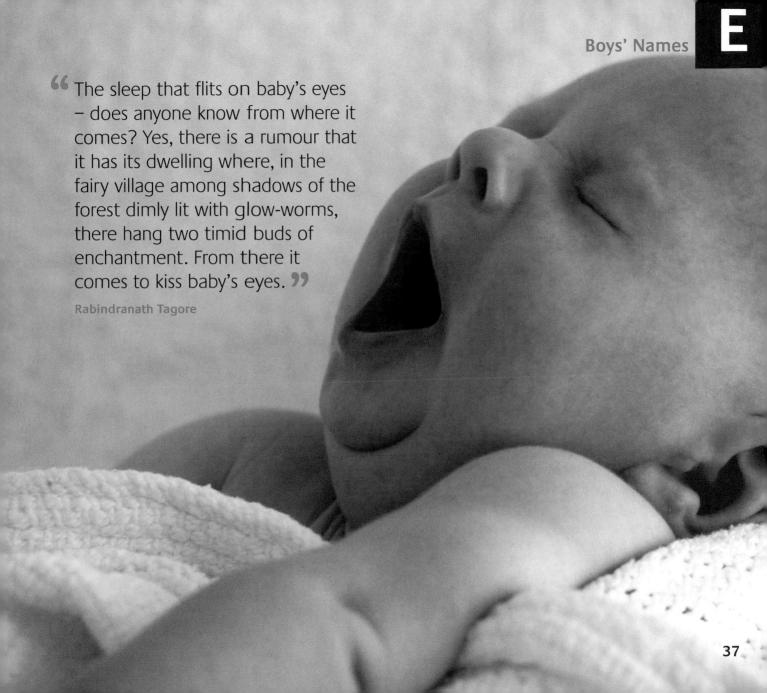

" The sleep that flits on baby's eyes – does anyone know from where it comes? Yes, there is a rumour that it has its dwelling where, in the fairy village among shadows of the forest dimly lit with glow-worms, there hang two timid buds of enchantment. From there it comes to kiss baby's eyes. "

Rabindranath Tagore

Boys' Names

Conquest. The revered St Edmund, 841–870, king of the East Angles, was defeated by the Danes in 870, and shot to death with arrows because he refused to renounce his Christianity.
Variations and abbreviations: Eamon (Ir), Ed, Eddie, Edmond (Fr), Edmondo (It), Edmundo (Sp), Ned, Nedely, Ted, Teddy.

Edward
Origin/meaning: Old English 'rich guardian'.
Like most names beginning with Ed- this is closely connected with the royal house of Wessex. Edward the Martyr, 963–978, succeeded his father King Edward and was murdered by his stepmother Elfrida. Edward the Confessor, 1003–1066, was the last of the Anglo-Saxon kings. He founded Westminster Abbey and was made a saint shortly after his death. Three Plantagenet kings, Edward I, Edward II and Edward III between them ruled England from 1272–1377, making the name an unshakeable favorite in England, and eventually in the rest of Europe. Five more English kings bore the name. After over a thousand years of use it is still popular today.
Variations and abbreviations: Duarte (Port), Ed, Eddie, Eddy, Edouard (Fr), Eduard (Ger/Dut), Eduardo (It/Port/Sp), Edvard (Scand), Ned, Neddie, Neddy, Ted, Teddie, Teddy.

Edwin
Origin/meaning: Old English 'rich friend'.
Edwin, King of Northumbria, 585–633, eventually gained overlordship over most of England. Northumbria at that time extended into Scotland and Edwin gave his name to Edinburgh. He was a convert to Christianity and was canonized after his death in battle.
Variations and abbreviations: Ed, Eddie, Eddy, Eduino (It/Sp), Edwyn, Ned, Neddie, Neddy, Odwin, Otwin, Ted, Teddie.

Elijah
Origin/meaning: Hebrew 'Jehovah is God'.
Elijah was a Hebrew Prophet who lived about 900 BC. He was fed by ravens at the brook Cherith and miraculously brought back to life the son of Zeraphath.

Elliot
Origin/meaning: Hebrew, Greek 'The Lord is my God'.
This widely-used name, especially in the US, comes from the same roots as Elias and Elijah q.v.
Variations: Eliot, Eliott, Elliott.

Ellis
Origin/meaning: Hebrew, Greek 'The Lord is my God'.
A last name that became a first name, Ellis comes from the same roots as Elijah q.v.

Elmer
Origin/meaning: Old English 'noble and famous'.
An English last name which developed from the Old English name Aylmer. It has been popular as a first name in the US, sometimes attributed to the Elmer brothers who were prominent in the American Revolution.

Elvis

Origin/meaning: Old Norse 'all wise'.
Recent use is almost totally due to the fame of the US singer Elvis Presley.

Emanuel

Origin/meaning: Hebrew 'God with us'.
A name used in the Old Testament to describe the promised Messiah (Isaiah ch.7 v.14). This is the Greek/Latin form of Immanuel. Its use in English-speaking countries has been confined mainly to Jewish people.
Variations and abbreviations: Emanuele (It), Emmanuel (Fr), Immanuel (Ger), Mannie, Manny, Manoel (Port), Manuel (Sp).

Emile

Origin/meaning: Latin: from the Roman clan name, Aemilius. Meaning sometimes given as 'zealous' or 'bronze beater'.
This is the masculine equivalent of Emily q.v. It is rare in English-speaking countries but frequently used in Germany and France.
Variations and abbreviations: Aemilius, Emil (Ger), Emilio (It/Sp), Emlyn (Wel).

Emlyn

Origin/meaning: Latin: from the Roman clan name, Aemilius. Meaning sometimes given as 'zealous' or 'bronze beater'.
This is the Welsh form of the name which is found in Europe as Emile or Emil.

Emrys

Origin/meaning: Greek 'divine' or 'immortal'.
The Welsh form of Ambrose q.v. Ambrosius Aurelianus was a legendary 5th-century Welsh king whose resistance to the Saxons may have given rise to the legends of King Arthur.

Enoch

Origin/meaning: uncertain. Possibly Hebrew 'mortal' or 'skilled'.
Enoch was a Hebrew patriarch, father of Methuselah (who was said to have lived 969 years) and grandfather of Noah (Genesis ch.5).
Variation: Enos (Greek).

Ephraim

Origin/meaning: uncertain. Sometimes given as Hebrew 'very fruitful'.
This is a Biblical name. Ephraim was the grandson of Jacob and gave his name to one of the tribes of Israel. It was used by 17th-century Puritans, particularly those living in New England.
Variations: Efrem, Ephraem, Ephrem.

Erasmus

Origin/meaning: Greek 'beloved'.
This name was used in the Netherlands and Germany in the Middle Ages. St Erasmus, a 4th-century martyr, was the patron saint

Boys' Names

of sailors. St Elmo's fire, an electrical discharge occurring round the masts of ships in a storm, was taken as a sign of the saint's protection. Desiderius Erasmus, 1466–1536, the eminent Dutch scholar and reformer spent much of his life in England.
Variations and abbreviations: Asmus, Elmo, Erasme (Fr), Erasmo (It), Telmo.

Eric

Origin/meaning: Old Norse usually given as 'ever ruling'.
This is a popular Scandinavian name and was brought to England and Scotland by the Scandinavian invaders who followed the fall of Roman rule. It was revived in England at the beginning of the 19th century because of the influence of the Romantic Movement.
Variations and abbreviations: Aic, Erich (Ger), Erick, Erico (It), Erik (Swed/Dan), Eirik (Nor), Jerik (Dan), Rick, Rickie, Ricky.

Ernest

Origin/meaning: Old German 'earnestness' or 'vigor'.
This was introduced into Britain in the 18th century by the Hanoverian royal family. Oscar Wilde used the name in his play 'The Importance of Being Earnest', 1895.
Variations and abbreviations: Earnest, Ern, Ernesto (It), Ernestin (Fr), Ernestus, Ernie.

Errol

Origin/meaning: Old English/Old Norse 'army power'.
A variation of the name Harold q.v. from one of its earliest forms, Eral. A popular US first name.

Esmé

Origin/meaning: French/Latin 'beloved'.
Used both as a masculine and a feminine name. Like the masculine Amyas it is a variation of the more popular Amy.
Variations: Aimé, Amyas.

Esmond

Origin/meaning: Old English 'grace protection'.
This Old English name had more or less died out as a first name by the end of the 14th century but survived as a comparatively unusual last name. In the 19th century, Thackeray's highly successful novel 'The History of Henry Esmond', 1852, brought the name back into currency as a personal name.

Ethan

Origin/meaning: Hebrew 'long-lived'.
This name's recent popularity is probably due in part to the actor Ethan Hawke, though it has been a widely-used name in the US for some time.

Etienne

Origin/meaning: Greek 'wreathed', 'crowned'.
A French form of Stephen q.v.

Euan/Ewan

Origin/meaning: Old Scots/Irish 'young warrior'.
This is probably from the same root as the common Welsh name Owen q.v.
Variations: Evan, Owain (Wel), Owen.

Eugene

Origin/meaning: Greek 'noble', 'well-born'.
This name was used in the Middle Ages to honor St Eugenius, a pope, but was popularized among the British and their allies by the exploits of Prince Eugene of Savoy, 1663–1736. He fought with them against the French, most notably with the Duke of Marlborough at Blenheim, 1704, Oudenarde, 1708 and Malplaquet, 1709. The name was popular in the US especially in its short form Gene.
Variations: Eugen (Ger), Eugène (Fr), Eugenio (It/Sp), Eugenius (Ger/Dut), Yevgeny (Rus).

Eustace

Origin/meaning: Greek 'fruitful'.
St Eustace was a Roman general. He was converted to Christianity while out hunting, by a vision of a stag with a luminous cross between its antlers. The soldier was later martyred and became one of the patron saints of huntsmen. The name came to England with the Normans.
Variations and abbreviations: Eustache (Fr), Eustachius (Ger), Eustasius (Ger/Dut), Eustatius (Dut), Eustazio (It), Eustic, Stacy.

Evan

Origin/meaning: Old Scots/Old Irish 'young warrior'.
An English form of the Scots name Euan q.v. and the Welsh names Owen q.v. and Ifan.

Evelyn (pron. Eevlyn)

Origin/meaning: diminutive of the Old German name Avi, or Old French 'hazel tree' or Old Celtic 'pleasant'.
Evelyn has been used as a masculine first name since the 16th century. It was used as a first name in families which had married into families with the last name Evelyn.

Everard

Origin/meaning: Old German 'strong as a boar'.
Introduced into England by the Normans.
Variations: Everett, Ewart.

Boys' Names

Ezra
Origin/meaning: Hebrew 'help'.
Ezra was a prophet who lived in the 5th century BC. His name was given to one of the Books of the Old Testament.
Variation: Esra (Ger).

F

Farquhar (pron. Fárkar)
Origin/meaning: Old Scots 'friendly man'.
This is used as a first name and, more commonly, as a last name in Scotland. Fearchur was an early Scottish king.

Felix
Origin/meaning: Latin 'fortunate'.
This is the name of over 50 saints, not all of whom are well documented. It is still used today although it is rather unusual.
Variations: Félicité (Fr), Félix (Fr), Felice, Feliciano (It).

Fergus
Origin/meaning: Old Irish/Old Scots 'choice of men'.
This is generally considered a Scottish name, although there is an Irish version. It gave rise to the Scottish last name Ferguson and is the name of ten saints.
Variations and abbreviations: Fergie, Feargus (Ir).

Finbar
Origin/meaning: Irish 'fair haired'.
A traditional Irish name that has recently become more widely used.
Variations: Finbarr, Fionnbharr.

Finlay
Origin/meaning: Scottish 'fair haired warrior'.
An old Scottish name, it has become more common in recent years.
Variation: Finley.

Fletcher
Origin/meaning: Old French 'arrow-maker'.
This is a family name sometimes used as a first name.

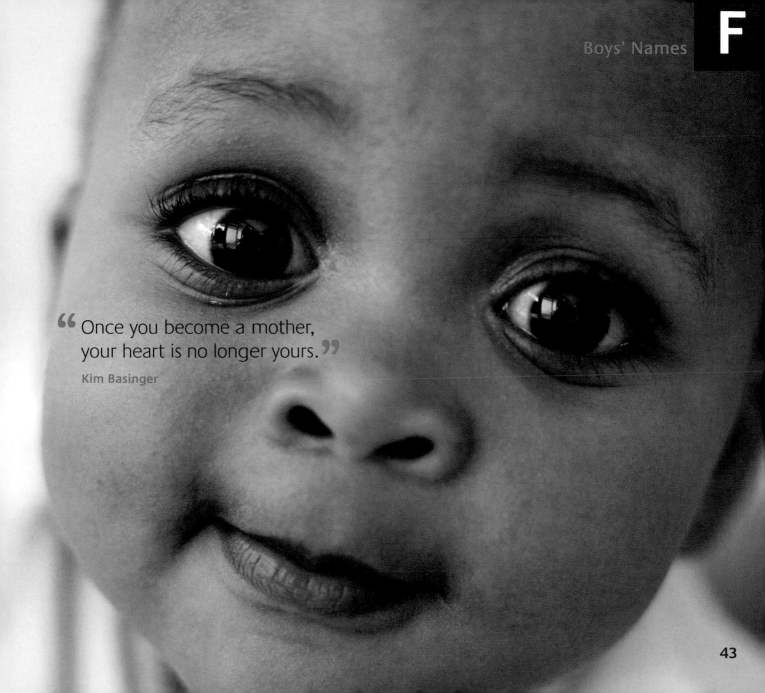

" Once you become a mother, your heart is no longer yours. "

Kim Basinger

F

Boys' Names

Floyd
Origin/meaning: Old Welsh 'grey'.
This is an English adaptation of the common Welsh name Lloyd. It is sometimes used as a first name derived from the family name.
Variation: Lloyd.

Forbes
Origin/meaning: Scottish 'field'.
Forbes is an old Scottish local name and last name that can now be found as a first name.

Ford
Origin/meaning: English 'ford'.
Though far better known as a last name Ford has achieved some popularity as a given name. Ford Maddox Ford's novel 'The Good Soldier', published in 1915, is regarded by many as one of the finest in the English language.

Francis
Origin/meaning: Old German 'a Frank'. Medieval Latin 'from France' or 'free'.
The Franks were a Teutonic race who took their name from the franca, a type of javelin. It was not until the 19th century that Francis became a popular English name. It is now used consistently in all English-speaking countries.
Variations and abbreviations: Chico (It), Ffransis (Wel), Fran, Francesco (It), Francisco (Sp/Port), François (Fr), Frank, Frankie, Frannie, Frans (Swed), Frants (Dan), Franz (Ger), Franziskus (Ger), Pancho (Sp).

Franklin
Origin/meaning: Old German 'a Frank'. Medieval English 'free citizen'.
The Frankish tribes prided themselves on their liberty and independence. Their name became a Latin word for free (francus) and Franklin, a diminutive of Frank, was the medieval word for a free man.
Variations and abbreviations: see Francis.

Franz
Origin/meaning: Old German 'a Frank' or 'free'.
A German familiar form of Francis (Franziscus) used frequently as an independent name.

Fraser
Origin/meaning: French 'strawberrier'.
This common Scottish last name comes from the Norman last name de Fresel, a place in France.
Variation: Frazer.

Fred
Origin/meaning: Old German 'peace'.
A short form of names beginning or ending with Fred, e.g. Frederick q.v. or Alfred q.v.

Frederick
Origin/meaning: Old English/Old German 'peace-rule'.
The -rick part of this name is the same word that is found in Richard and in words like rex (the Latin word for king), and reich (the German word for kingdom).
Variations and abbreviations: Federico (It), Federigo (Sp), Ferry (Med Eng), Fred, Freddie, Freddy, Frédéric (Fr), Frederic, Frederich, Frederik (Dan/Dut), Fredric, Fredrick, Friedrich (Ger), Fritz (Ger), Rick, Rickie, Ricky, Rik.

Frodo
Origin/meaning: Old Norse 'wise'.
This is the invented name of the hero of the epic novel and film trilogy 'The Lord of the Rings'. However, there is a real Scandinavian name Frode.

G

Gabriel
Origin/meaning: Hebrew 'strong man of God'.
Gabriel, with Michael and Raphael is one of the three archangels named in the Bible. He was the one chosen to announce the coming birth of John the Baptist to his father, Zacharias the Priest, and to announce to the Virgin Mary the coming birth of Christ.
Variations and abbreviations: Gabby, Gabe, Gabriele (It), Gavrilo (Russ).

Galahad
Origin/meaning: uncertain. Usually given as Welsh 'battle hawk' to tie in with the similar Gawain q.v.
Sir Galahad was the son of Elaine and Sir Lancelot. He grew up to be the only knight pure enough in thought and deed to successfully complete the search for the Holy Grail.
Variation: Galaad.

Ganesh (pron. Ganess)
Origin/meaning: Sanskrit 'head of the Ganas'. (The Ganas are demi-gods who wait on Shiva.)
This is a very popular name in India because the god it honors is the god of wisdom and patron of the arts, more or less the equivalent of the Greek goddess Athena.
Variations: Ganapati, Ganesha.

Boys' Names

Gareth

Origin/meaning: either Old German 'hard-spear' (from Gerard) or Welsh 'gentle'.
Gareth is yet another character from the tales of King Arthur and his Knights of the Round Table. Tennyson used it for 'Gareth and Lynnet', 1872, in one of the episodes of his 'Idylls of the King'.
Variations and abbreviations: Garrett, Garth, Gary, Gerard.

Garth

Origin/meaning: Welsh 'high-land' or a form of Gareth q.v.
This is the name of several mountains in Wales and is used as a Welsh name. It may also be a modern short form of Gareth q.v. It was the name of a comic strip hero who appeared for many years in the 'Daily Mirror'.

Gary

Origin/meaning: Old German 'spear'.
A short form of Gerald and Gerard q.v. through the form Garret. Also used as a form of Gareth q.v.

Gavin

Origin/meaning: uncertain. Usually given as Welsh 'hawk of the plain'.
A medieval form of Gawain q.v.

Gawain

Origin/meaning: uncertain. Usually given as Welsh 'hawk of the plain' or 'little hawk'. Possibly also Old German 'tribute' or 'partition of land'.
Sir Gawain is one of the characters in the Tales of King Arthur and his Knights of the Round Table. He was nicknamed 'the courteous', and is famous for his encounter with the Green Knight.
Variations: Gauvaine, Gavin, Gawayne, Gawen, Gawin, Gwion.

Gaylord

Origin/meaning: Old French 'merry', 'high-spirited'.
This is derived from the French word gaillard. In the US it has become an established first name.

Gene

Origin/meaning: Greek 'noble', 'well-born'.
This is the usual short form of Eugene q.v. in the US, where it is frequently found as an independent name.
Variations and abbreviations: see Eugene.

Geoffrey

Origin/meaning: Old German. Uncertain. Probably 'district peace'. Sometimes given as 'traveler peace'.
A common medieval name. The alternative spelling is Jeffrey. Its early popularity is evident from the many last names such as Jeffreys, Jepherson and Jeeves, which derive from it.
Variations and abbreviations: Geoff, Geoffroi (Fr), Geoffroy (Fr), Jeff, Jeffrey.

George

Origin/meaning: Greek 'farmer'.

St George was a Roman officer martyred at Lydda in 303 for his adherence to the Christian faith. He is the patron saint of Greece as well as England and the centre of his cult was in Palestine where he was martyred. Crusaders, returning from the Holy Land, introduced it to England. In 1349 Edward III dedicated his new Order of the Garter to St George, thus designating him as the patron saint of England. On the accession of the Hanoverian King George I in 1714 the name started to become generally popular. By 1830 when George IV died there had been a George on the British throne for 116 years, and it had become a standard name.

Variations and abbreviations: Dod, Doddy, Geordie, Georg (Ger), Georges (Fr), Georgie, Georgy, Giorgio (It), Jöran (Swed), Jorge (Sp), Jörgen (Dan), Seiorse (Ir), Siôr (Wel), Yorick, Yuri (Russ).

Geraint (pron. Gerrighnt or Jerrighnt)

Origin/meaning: Greek 'old'.

Like several other Welsh names this is based on a Roman name. The original is probably the Roman name Gerontius. The name is found in the collection of Welsh Celtic tales, 'The Mabinogion', and Tennyson used the tale of 'Enis and Geraint' as one of the episodes in his 'Idylls of the King', 1859.

Gerald

Origin/meaning: Old German 'spear-rule'.

This name was adopted by the Normans who introduced it into England. It is sometimes confused with Gerard q.v. which is similar in meaning and origin.

Variations and abbreviations: Gary, Gearalt (Ir), Gerallt (Wel), Géralde (Fr), Gerold (Ger), Gerrie, Gerry, Giraldo (It), Giraud (Fr), Jerold, Jerrie, Jerry.

Gerard

Origin/meaning: Old German 'spear-hard'.

This is a similar name to Gerald and was more popular in the Middle Ages, giving rise to several last names including Garrard and Garret.

Variations and abbreviations: Gary, Garry, Garret, Gearard (Ir), Geraud (Fr), Gerardo (Sp/It), Gerhard (Ger/Scand), Gerhardt (Ger), Gerrard, Gearoid, Gerry, Jerry.

Gershom

Origin/meaning: Hebrew 'bell'. Sometimes given as 'stranger'.

A Biblical name given to the first born child of Moses and Zipporah. Nowadays it is used mainly by Jewish people.

Variation: Gersham.

Gervase

Origin/meaning: uncertain. Possibly Old German 'spear' plus Celtic 'servant' (as in vassal).

St Gervase was an early martyr.

Variations: Gervais, Gervaise (Fr), Gervasio (It), Gervaso (It), Gervasius (Ger), Jaruis.

G

Boys' Names

Gideon
Origin/meaning: Hebrew 'destroyer', 'tree feller'.
A Biblical name of one of the Judges of Israel.
Variations: Gedeon, Gédéon (Fr), Gedeone (It).

Gilbert
Origin/meaning: Old German 'bright pledge'.
The Normans introduced this name into England and it was a great favorite in the Middle Ages. St Gilbert of Sempringham, 1085–1189, was the founder of the only English religious order, the Gilbertines.
Variations and abbreviations: Bert, Bertie, Berty, Gib, Gibb, Gil, Gilberto (It), Gilbrecht (Ger), Gill, Giselbert (Ger), Giselbrecht (Ger).

Giles
Origin/meaning: uncertain. Usually given as Greek 'kid' therefore 'youthful'.
The Latin name Aegidius was said to be taken from the Greek word for kid. The name reached France, probably before the 9th century, because of St Aegidius (a Greek hermit so named because he wore a goat skin) who settled in France. The French adapted the name to Gide, then Gilles, which is the form in which it reached England in the 12th century. St Gilles (Aegidius) saved the life of his pet hind, which was being hunted, by taking it in his arms and being shot himself.
Variations and abbreviations: Aegidius, Egide (Fr), Egidio (It), Egidius (Dut), Gide, Gil (Sp/Ger), Gill (Ger), Gilles (Fr), Gyles.

Giorgio
Origin/meaning: Greek 'farmer'.
A prevalent Italian form of George, for example, the fashion designer Giorgio Armani.

Glenn
Origin/meaning: Celtic 'valley', 'glen'.
It probably began in the US as a family name used as a first name. It has also been used to honor John Glenn, the American astronaut.
Variations: Glen, Glyn (Wel), Glynn.

Glyn
Origin/meaning: Welsh 'valley' or possibly a short form of Glyndwr (Glendower).
A popular Welsh name now also fairly common outside Wales.
Variations: Glenn (Scot/Ir), Glynn.

Godfrey
Origin/meaning: Old German/Old English 'God's peace'.
Introduced by the Normans in the 11th century.
Variations: Godefroi (Fr), Godofredo (Sp), Golfredo (It), Gottfrid (Scand), Gottfried (Ger).

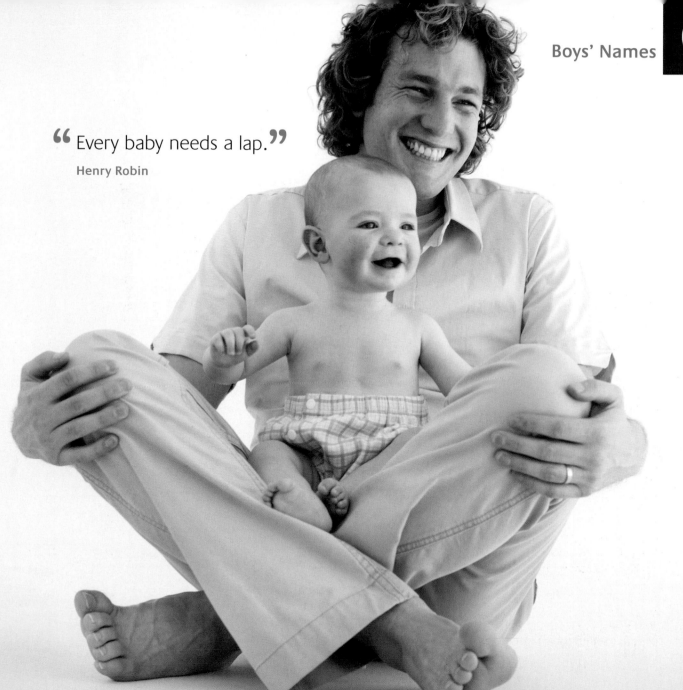

66 Every baby needs a lap. **99**

Henry Robin

Boys' Names

Gordon
Origin/meaning: uncertain. Possibly Scots Gaelic 'by the great hill'.
The name of one of a famous Scottish clan, the Gordons. In Britain it was often given to honor General Gordon, 1833–1885, who died defending Khartoum against the troops of the Mahdi.
Variations and abbreviations: Gorden, Gordie, Gordy.

Goronwy (pron. Gorónwee)
Origin/meaning: Welsh 'hero'.
A popular Welsh first name.
Variations and abbreviations: Gronow, Gronw, Ronw.

Graham
Origin/meaning: Old English 'gravelly homestead' or 'from Grantham'.
This name was taken to Scotland in the Middle Ages by an Anglo-Norman nobleman. It came into use as a first name in the 19th century.
Variations and abbreviations: Graeme, Grahame, Grame.

Grant
Origin/meaning: French 'tall'.
This is a last name which came into use as a first name in the 19th century. In the US it was used to honor General Ulysses S. Grant, 1822–1885, the 18th President and hero of the Civil War.

Gregory
Origin/meaning: Greek 'watchman'.
A name which has many associations with the Orthodox and Catholic churches. In the Western church there were sixteen Pope Gregorys. The best known in England is the first, St Gregory the Great, 540–604, who sent St Augustine to England to convert the Anglo-Saxons.
Variations and abbreviations: Greer (Eng), Greg, Gregg, Grégoire (Fr), Gregor (Scot/Ger), Greggor (Dut), Gregorio (Sp/It), Gregorius (Dut/Ger), Grigori (Russ).

Griffith
Origin/meaning: Old Welsh 'lord'.
This is the English spelling of the Welsh Gruffudd. Often found as a last name outside Wales, it has also become usual as a first name.
Variations and abbreviations: Griff, Griffin.

Guy
Origin/meaning: Old German, uncertain, possibly 'wood' or 'wild'.

Guy, Earl of Warwick was a legendary hero of the Middle Ages, in love with Phelis the Fair. He had to succeed in many doughty deeds to win her hand. The attempt by Guy Fawkes to blow up James I in the Houses of Parliament placed the name firmly out of fashion in Britain. In the 19th century it was reintroduced by writers of the Romantic Movement such as Sir Walter Scott in his novel 'Guy Mannering', 1815.
Variations and abbreviations: Guido (Fr/Ger/It/Sp), Vito (It), Vitas, Wido (Ger).

Gwilym
Origin/meaning: Old German 'helmet of resolution'.
The Welsh form of William q.v.

Gwyn
Origin/meaning: Welsh 'white/fair' or 'good'.
A short form of names like Gwynfor or an independent name.
Variations: Gwynn, Gwynne, Wynne.

H

Habib
Origin/meaning: Arabic 'beloved'.
A name found in all Muslim countries.

Hal
Origin/meaning: Old German 'home-ruler'.
This was the most usual pet form of Henry for many hundreds of years. King Henry VIII was known to his people as Good King Hal.
Variations and abbreviations: see Henry.

Hamish
Origin/meaning: uncertain. Usually given as 'supplanter'.
The English spelling of Seumas, the Scottish form of James q.v.
Variations and abbreviations: see James.

Hanif
Origin/meaning: Arabic 'true believer'.
This is a Muslim name, found in North Africa.

Boys' Names

Hank
Origin/meaning: Old German 'home ruler'.
A familiar form of Henry confined almost entirely to the US.
Variations and abbreviations: see Henry.

Harold
Origin/meaning: Old English/Old Norse 'army power'.
After King Harold was killed by William the Conqueror's invaders at the battle of Hastings the name died out in England.
It survived successfully in its other native land, Norway, where three kings bore the name. When old names were revived in the
19th century, Harold reappeared.
Variations and abbreviations: Araldo (It), Errol (Eng), Harald (Scand), Harry, Herold (Dut).

Haroun
Origin/meaning: Arabic 'exalted'.
A common Muslim name in North Africa.
Variation: Harun.

Harrison
Origin/meaning: English 'son of Harry'.
A last name that has become much used as a first name thanks to the fame of Hollywood actor Harrison Ford.
Variation and abbreviation: Harry.

Harry
Origin/meaning: Old German: 'home-ruler'.
In the last 100 years this has been used as a familiar form of Henry and in the last few years Harry has again been used in England
as an independent name and not as a pet name. The wide use of the name can be deduced from the expression 'every Tom,
Dick and Harry' meaning everybody.
Variations and abbreviations: see Henry.

Harvey
Origin/meaning: Celtic French 'battle worthy' or Old German 'warrior in battle'.
This is a name introduced by the Normans, but is similar to the Saxon name Harvig. Harvey developed most successfully as a last
name. In the 19th century it was one of many last names which were revived as first names.
Variations: Herve (Fr), Hervey, Herwig (Ger).

Hasan
Origin/meaning: Arabic 'handsome'.
A version of this name is found in all Muslim countries.
Variations: Hasani, Husani (E Africa).

Hayden

Origin/meaning: English 'hedged valley'.
More common as a last name, but now often used as a given name as well.
Variations: Haden, Hadyn.

Hector

Origin/meaning: Greek 'steadfast'.
Hector was a Trojan hero, the son of Priam and Hecuba. He was killed by the Greek Achilles, who added insult to injury by dragging his body three times round the walls of Troy.
Variations: Ector (Fr), Ettore (It).

Henry

Origin/meaning: Old German 'home-ruler'.
This name was introduced into England by the Normans in the form Henri. In England Henry and Harry developed simultaneously but although Harry was probably more used, Henry is usually assumed to be the slightly more formal version.
Variations and abbreviations: Arrigo (It), Enrico (It), Enrique (Sp), Hal, Hank, Harry, Heindrick, Heinrich (Ger), Heinz (Ger), Hendrik (Dut/Scand), Henne (Scand), Henri (Fr), Henrik (Scand).

Herbert

Origin/meaning: Old English/Old German 'bright army'.
This Saxon name was a favorite of the Normans who brought over their own version of it after the Conquest. Like many early names it was rediscovered in the 19th century. Its popularity was also aided by the fact that Herbert was the aristocratic last name of a family which had arrived with the Conqueror.
Variations and abbreviations: Aribert (Fr), Ariberto (It), Bert, Bertie, Berty, Erberto (It), Harbert, Haribert, Hebert, Herb, Herbiberto (Sp), Herbie.

Hew

Origin/meaning: Old German 'understanding' or 'thought'.
A form of Hugh q.v.

Hilary

Origin/meaning: Medieval Latin 'cheerful'.
The masculine and feminine forms of this medieval name are the same. The feast day of St Hilary (Hilaire) of Poitiers, 315–367, is January 14th and because of this the first law and university term of the calendar year became known as the Hilary term in the UK.
Variations: Hilaire (Fr), Hilar (Ger), Hilario (Sp/Port), Hilarius (Dut/Ger/Scand), Ilario (It).

Hiram

Origin/meaning: uncertain. Sometimes given as Hebrew 'my brother is high'.

Boys' Names

Hiram was the king of Tyre, the Lebanese sea-port. Lebanon was famous for its cedars which Hiram supplied to King David and King Solomon, to build the temple in Jerusalem.
Abbreviations: Hi, Hy.

Homer
Origin/meaning: Greek 'pledge' or 'hostage'.
The name of the Greek epic poet, author of the 'Odyssey' and the 'Iliad', is occasionally used as a first name.
Variations: Homère (Fr), Homerus (Dut/Ger), Omero (It).

Horace
Origin/meaning: Latin, from Horatius, the name of a famous Roman clan.
This French form of Horatius became an alternative form of the name in England, together with Horatio.

Horatio (pron. Horáysheeo)
Origin/meaning: Latin, from Horatius, the name of a famous Roman clan.
Horatio probably arrived in England from Italy in about the 16th century. Shakespeare has a character called Horatio in his play 'Hamlet', 1600. The Roman family produced many remarkable people, including Publius Horatius Cocles, a hero who defended single-handed the bridge across the Tiber into Rome against the invading Etruscans. Admiral Nelson, 1758–1805, the hero of the Battle of Trafalgar, was named Horatio after his godfather.
Variations and abbreviations: Hod, Horace (Fr/Eng), Horacid (Sp/Port), Horas, Horatius, Horaz (Ger), Horry, Orazio (It).

Howard
Origin/meaning: either Old German 'brave thought' or Middle English 'hayward' (the guardian of the animal enclosure).
This name developed in the Middle Ages into a last name, most notably of the Earls of Norfolk, hereditary Earls Marshal of England.
Variations and abbreviations: Howey, Howie.

Hubert
Origin/meaning: Old German/Old English 'bright thought'.
A popular medieval name, perhaps because of St Hubert, d.727, who, according to legend, was converted to Christianity by finding a stag with a cross between its antlers.
Variations and abbreviations: Bert, Bertie, Berty, Hubertus (Dut/Ger), Huberto (Sp/It), Hugbert (Ger), Oberto (It), Uberto (It).

Hugh
Origin/meaning: Old German 'understanding' or 'thought'.
This was a name introduced by the Normans into Britain, although a similar Celtic name, Huw q.v. already existed. The English Hugh is pronounced like the Medieval French but the spelling reflects the German/Latin Hugo.
Variations: Hew, Huey, Hughie, Hugo (Ger/Latin), Hughes (Fr), Huw (Wel), Ugo (It).

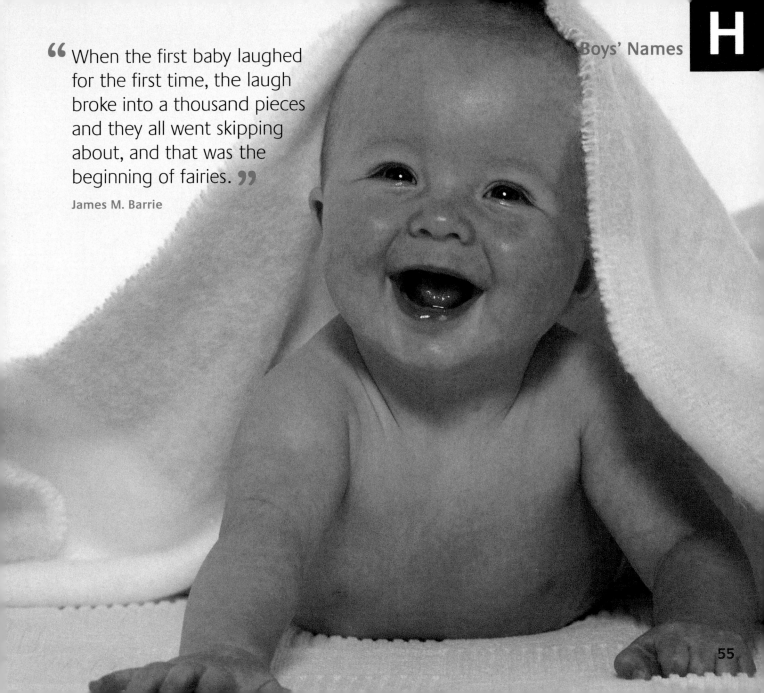

" When the first baby laughed for the first time, the laugh broke into a thousand pieces and they all went skipping about, and that was the beginning of fairies. "

James M. Barrie

Boys' Names

Hugo
Origin/meaning: Old German 'understanding' or 'thought'.
This German Latin form of Hugh was used in England in the Middle Ages and is coming back into favor.

Hunter
Origin/meaning: English 'hunter'.
An old occupational last name that became well known as a first name thanks to the controversial American journalist and writer Hunter S. Thompson.

Huw
Origin/meaning: Celtic 'fire'.
This Welsh name is now usually assumed to be the same as the Old German Hugh q.v. although their origins and meanings are really separate.

Hyman
Origin/meaning: Hebrew 'life'.
This is primarily a Jewish name. It is the English form of Chaim.
Variations and abbreviations: Chaim, Hayyim, Hy, Hymie, Mannie, Manny.

Hywel (pron. Howell)
Origin/meaning: Welsh 'eminent'.
A popular Welsh first name. Hywel Dda (Hywel the Good), d.950, was one of the most famous Welsh Kings. During his reign Welsh law was first codified. Hywel has given rise to several last names. One of these, Powell, is a contraction of Ap Hywel, which means son of Hywel.
Variations: Hoel (Celtic Fr), Howel (Eng), Howell (Eng), Powell.

I

Iago
Origin/meaning: uncertain. Possible Hebrew 'supplant'.
The Spanish and Welsh form of Jacob/James q.v. from the Latin version Jacobus. Iago causes the destruction of Othello in Shakespeare's play.

Iain/Ian
Origin/meaning: Hebrew 'Jehovah has favored'.

The Scots form of John. Iain is regarded as the slightly more authentic spelling and is the version still found mainly in Scotland.
Variations and abbreviations: see John.

Idris

Origin/meaning: Old Welsh 'fiery lord'.
Id- is a part of many Welsh names and it means lord. Idris is one of the most popular Welsh names but it does not have an English form. In Welsh legend Idris Gawr (the giant) was a magician, philosopher and astronomer who had his observatory on the mountain Cader Idris (seat of Idris).

Ifor (pron. Eevor)

Origin/meaning: Old Celtic 'lord'.
A name related to other Welsh names beginning with Id- or ending with -udd, both of which mean lord in Welsh. The Cornish saint Ifor gave his name to the little town of Saint Ives.
Variations and abbreviations: Ifar, Ives, Ivor (Eng).

Ignatius

Origin/meaning: uncertain. Possibly Latin 'fiery'.
This was originally a Greek name which may have been interpreted as fiery because of the similarity to the Latin word 'ignis' – 'fire'. In the Eastern Church it was popular because of St Ignatius, Bishop of Antioch who was martyred about AD 114. The name also belonged to a vigorous leader of the counter-reformation St Ignatius Loyola, the founder of the Jesuits.
Variations and abbreviations: Enesco, Enego, Ignace (Fr), Ignacio (Sp), Ignaz (Ger), Ignazio (It), Inigo.

Imran

Origin/meaning: Arabic 'strong'.
A well-known Muslim name in Britain thanks to the great Pakistani cricket all-rounder Imran Khan.

Indiana

Origin/meaning: English 'land of the Indians'.
The name of a US state, Indiana has become used as a first name thanks to the fictional character Indiana Jones played in a series of Hollywood films by Harrison Ford.
Variation and abbreviation: Indy.

Ingmar

Origin/meaning: Old Norse/Old German 'famous Ingvi'.
A Scandinavian name, one of many containing the name of the hero-god Ing or Ingvi. He was a hero of the Teutonic (Germanic) tribes who spread throughout Northern Europe including Britain. He may have given his name to the Angles who were one of the tribes which invaded Britain, and he therefore may be the source of the name England.
Variations and abbreviations: Ingemar, Ingo.

I

Boys' Names

Inigo
Origin/meaning: uncertain. Possibly Latin 'fiery'.
A form of Ignatius q.v. familiar because of the first great English architect Inigo Jones, 1573–1652, who introduced the Palladian style of architecture into England.

Iolo
Origin/meaning: uncertain, possibly Greek 'downy', i.e. 'unbearded', 'youthful'.
Commonly assumed to be the Welsh form of Julius.

Irving
Origin/meaning: uncertain. Possibly Old English 'sea friend' or 'green river'.
A last name derived from an English place-name. It has become a popular 20th-century first name in the US, particularly among Jewish people.

Isaac
Origin/meaning: uncertain. Possibly a non-Hebrew name. Usually given as Hebrew 'laughter'.
Abraham's wife Sarah was past the age of child-bearing when she gave birth to Isaac her first child. The name is usually supposed to refer to her laughter of joy.
Variations and abbreviations: Ike, Ikey, Isaak (Ger/Dut), Isacco (It), Izak, Izaak.

Ivan
Origin/meaning: Hebrew 'Jehovah has favored'.
The Russian form of John q.v. used by six notable Russian Grand Dukes and Tsars.
Variations and abbreviations: see John.

Ivor
Origin/meaning: Old Welsh 'lord'.
The English version of the Welsh Ifor q.v. a name found, in several forms, in all Celtic areas.
Variations: Ifar (Wel), Ifor (Wel), Ivar, Iver, Ives, Yvor.

J

Jack
Origin/meaning: Hebrew 'Jehovah has favored'.
This is a long established familiar form of John from the medieval form Jankin. In the 20th century it has been much used as an independent name.
Variations and abbreviations: Jackie, Jacko (Scot), Jacky.

Jacob

Origin/meaning: uncertain. Possibly Hebrew 'supplanter'.
Both James and Jacob come from the same Hebrew name Aqob. The patriarch Jacob tricked his father Isaac into giving him the elder son's blessing intended for Esau.
Variations and abbreviations: Cob, Cobb, Giacobbe (It), Giacobo (It), Giacopo (It), Jacobo (Sp), Jake, Jakie, Jakob (Ger).

Jackson

Origin/meaning: English 'son of Jack'.
Though best known as a last name, it is used in the US as a given name.

Jake

Origin/meaning: uncertain. Possibly Hebrew 'supplanter'.
A Medieval English form of Jacob/James possibly from the French form Jacques, which the English pronounced Jakes.
Variation: Jaikie.

James

Origin/meaning: Possibly Hebrew 'supplanter'.
James is a form of the Hebrew name Aqob. It was brought back by pilgrims who had visited the famous shrine at Compostella in Spain where the remains of the apostle St James the Great were said to be buried. By the 13th century it was a well-established name in England and also in Scotland, where it was the name of seven kings. The accession in 1603 of one of these, James I, in succession to Queen Elizabeth, brought about a period of great popularity for the name.
Variations and abbreviations: Diego (Sp), Giacomo (It), Hamish (Anglo-Scot), Iago (Sp/Wel), Jacques (Fr), Jago (Cornish), Jaime (Sp), Jake, Jamey, Jamie, Jay, Jayme (Sp), Jem, Jemmy, Jim, Jimi, Jimmie, Jimmy, Seamus (Ir), Seumas (Scot), Shamus (Anglo-Ir).

Jamie

Origin/meaning: uncertain. Possibly Hebrew 'supplanter'.
A Scottish familiar form of James q.v.

Jarvis

Origin/meaning: Old German 'spear' plus Celtic 'servant'.
A form of Gervase q.v. usually found as a last name but sometimes used as a first name.

Jason

Origin/meaning: uncertain. Sometimes given as Greek 'healer'.
This is a Biblical name, which came into use in the 17th century. It is a rendering of the name Eason which occurs in Acts 17 vs.5–9 and St Paul's Epistle to the Romans ch.16. The English form was presumably influenced by the name of Jason the Greek mythological hero.

J

Boys' Names

Jasper
Origin/meaning: uncertain. Possibly Persian. Sometimes given as 'treasurer' because of the legend of the three wise men. The names traditionally given to the three wise men who brought gifts to the infant Jesus are Caspar, Melchior and Balthazar. These names became current in the Middle Ages, although they do not appear in the Bible. Jasper is the English version of Caspar q.v.
Variations: Caspar, Gaspar (Sp), Gaspard (Fr), Gaspare (It), Jesper (Scand).

Javed
Origin/meaning: Arabic 'immortal'.
The former Pakistan cricket captain Javed Miandad helped make this name more common.

Jay
Origin/meaning: Old French 'jay'.
The name of this common European bird has been used as an English last name since the Middle Ages. It may have been applied initially to someone with either the jay's beauty or its characteristic of endless chattering. In the 20th century it has been used, mainly in the US, as a first name. Jay is sometimes used as a short form of names beginning with the letter J.

Jayden
Origin/meaning: Hebrew 'God has heard'.
Popular in the US.
Variation: Jaden.

Jed
Origin/meaning: Hebrew 'beloved of the Lord'.
This is a short form of the Biblical name Jedidiah, a name used for King Solomon. The original is now obsolete, but Jed has become quite a common independent name in the US.

Jeevan
Origin/meaning: Sanskrit 'life'.
A popular name in India.

Jefferson
Origin/meaning: English 'son of Jeffrey'.
The name is sometimes given in honor of the great statesman and 3rd US president Thomas Jefferson, 1743–1826.

Jeffrey
Origin/meaning: uncertain. Probably Old German 'district peace'. Sometimes given as 'traveler peace'. An alternative spelling of Geoffrey q.v. a common medieval name which is again popular today.

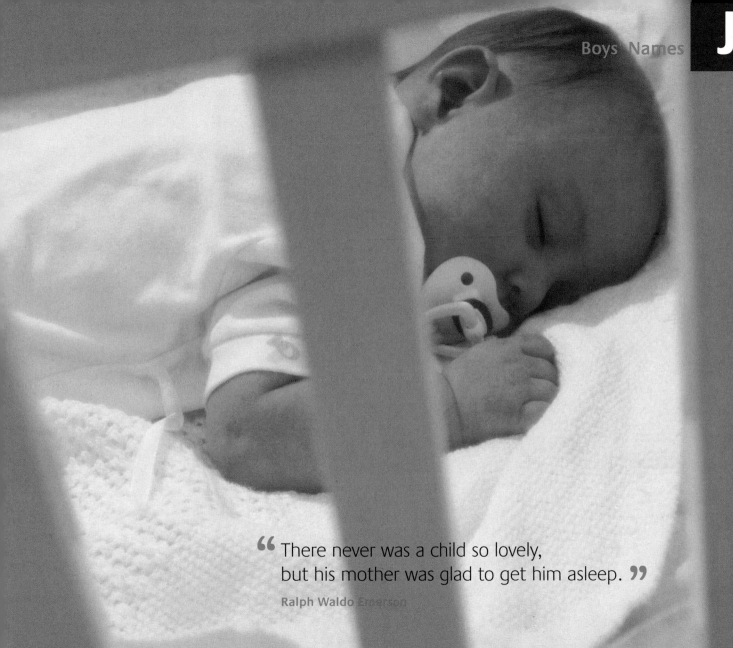

"There never was a child so lovely,
but his mother was glad to get him asleep. "
Ralph Waldo Emerson

J

Boys' Names

Jehangir
Origin/meaning: Sanskrit 'conqueror of the world'.
A Muslim name. Jehangir, 1569–1627, was the third Mogul Emperor of India. His father was Akbar. His real interests were literature and art and it was he who laid out the famous Shalimar gardens in Kashmir. During his reign the government was effectively run by Nur Jehan q.v. his remarkable wife.
Variation: Jahangir.

Jem
Origin/meaning: uncertain. Possibly Hebrew 'supplanter'.
An old short form of James from a medieval form Jeames. It has now been superseded by the more modern Jim/Jimmy.
Variation: Jemmy. See also James.

Jeremy
Origin/meaning: Hebrew 'God is high'.
This is the native English form of the name of the prophet Jeremiah. It developed in the Middle Ages from the Greek/Latin Jeremias.
Variations and abbreviations: see Jeremiah.

Jermyn
Origin/meaning: Latin 'a German'.

Jerome
Origin/meaning: Greek 'sacred name'.
Jerome is the English form of the Greek name Hieronymous. This became an acceptable Christian name in the Middle Ages because of St Eusebius Sophronius Hieronymous, 342–420, known in England as St Jerome. He was an ascetic and one of the greatest Biblical scholars.
Variations and abbreviations: Gerome, Geronimo (It), Gerrie, Gerry, Hieronymous (Dut/Ger), Jérôme (Fr), Jerry.

Jesse (pron. Jessy)
Origin/meaning: Hebrew 'Jehovah exists'.
This is a Biblical name brought into general use after the Reformation. Jesse was the father of King David and therefore the first in the direct family tree of Jesus Christ.
Variations and abbreviations: Jess, Jessie.

Jethro
Origin/meaning: Hebrew 'pre-eminence'.
This Hebrew name may well have begun as a title (cf. English names Earl and Prince). The name is found in the Old Testament as the father-in-law of Moses.

Jevan
Origin/meaning: Hebrew 'Jehovah has favored'.
This is one of several Anglo-Welsh forms of John. The true native Welsh form of John is Siôn.
Variations: Evan, Owen.

Jim
Origin/meaning: uncertain. Possibly Hebrew 'supplanter'.
The most usual modern short form of James q.v.
Variations: Jimi, Jimmie, Jimmy. See also James.

Jocelyn
Origin/meaning: Old German 'a man of the Goths'.
Jocelyn was one of many Teutonic names brought to England by the Normans and in the Middle Ages Jocelyn was not an unusual name. In the 20th century it tends to be given in families where it has become traditional.
Variations: Jocelin, Joscelin, Joss.

Joe
Origin/meaning: Hebrew 'May Jehovah increase'.
The usual English short form of Joseph q.v. Sometimes used as an independent name.
Variations: Jo, Joey. See also Joseph.

Joel
Origin/meaning: Hebrew 'Jehovah is God'.
A Biblical name. Joel was a minor Hebrew prophet in the 5th century BC. A Book of the Old Testament contains his prophecies.

John
Origin/meaning: Hebrew 'Jehovah has favored' (via the Latin form Johannes).
An important Christian name since almost a hundred early saints were called John. Chief among them were of course St John the Baptist and St John the Evangelist. Initially a popular name in the area of the Eastern Orthodox Church, it was popularized in Western Europe by returning Crusaders. It has equivalents in every European language.
Variations and abbreviations: Evan (Anglo-Wel), Ewan (Anglo-Scot), Ewen, Giovanni (It), Hans (Ger), Iain (Scot), Ian, Jack, Jacky, Jan (Dut/Slav), Janesi, Jean (Fr), Jens (Dan), Jevan (Anglo-Wel), Jock (Scot), Jocko, Johan, Johann, Johannes (Ger), Johnnie, Johnny, Jon, Jonn, Juan (Sp), Owen (Anglo-Wel), Sean (Ir), Shaughn (Ir), Shaun, Shawn (Anglo-Ir), Siôn (Wel), Zane.

Jolyon
Origin/meaning: from the Roman family name Julius possibly meaning 'downy'.
A north country English form of Julian given wider currency by John Galsworthy (1867–1933) in his novel sequence 'The Forsyte Saga', 1920–1934.

Boys' Names

Jon
Origin/meaning: Hebrew 'Jehovah has favored' or Hebrew 'Jehovah gave'.
A short form of either John or Jonathan.

Jonah
Origin/meaning: Hebrew 'dove'.
Jonah was the name of a Hebrew prophet. God told him to go to Ninevah and prophesy but he grew frightened and fled by ship. God caused the ship to be wrecked and the enraged sailors threw Jonah into the sea where he was swallowed by a large fish and eventually cast out onto land.
Variation: Jonas.

Jonathan
Origin/meaning: Hebrew 'Jehovah gave'.
Jonathan is sometimes confused with the separate name John q.v. as they share the short form Jon. Jonathan was the son of Saul and friend of David. The expression 'a David and Jonathan' means two inseparable friends.
Variations and abbreviations: Gionata (It), Jon, Jonathon, Jonty. See also Nathaniel, Theodore.

Jordan
Origin/meaning: Hebrew 'flowing down'.
Jordan has been used as a masculine and feminine name since the Crusaders brought back the name of this river from the Holy Land in the Middle Ages.

Joseph
Origin/meaning: Hebrew 'may Jehovah increase'.
Joseph was the favorite son of Jacob and Rachel whose brothers, envying the coat of many colors which was a sign of their father's favor, sold him into captivity in Egypt. Joseph was also used in the Middle Ages as a Christian name to honor St Joseph, the husband of the Blessed Virgin Mary, and St Joseph of Arimathea who provided the tomb for Jesus. It was Joseph of Arimathea who is traditionally supposed to have come to England and built a church at Glastonbury.
Variations and abbreviations: Beppo (It), Giuseppe (It), Iossif (Russ), Iossip (Russ), Jo, Joe, Joey, José (Sp), Josef (Ger), Josephus.

Joshua
Origin/meaning: Hebrew 'Jehovah saves'.
Joshua was the successor of Moses. Joshua was much loved as a name by Puritans on both sides of the Atlantic in the 17th and 18th centuries.
Variations and abbreviations: Giosué (It), Josh, Josua (Ger), Josué (Fr).

Jude
Origin/meaning: Hebrew 'praise of the Lord'.

The Anglicized form of the Jewish name Judah.
Variations and abbreviations: Jud, Judah, Judas, Judd, Yehudi.

Julian

Origin/meaning: from Julius, a Roman family name, possibly meaning 'downy'.
Julian's popularity was due in part to the great number of saints who bore the name. The most popular of these was Julian the Hospitaler. He was said to have accidentally killed his parents and in expiation went to live by a ford where he and his wife helped poor travelers, one of whom was Christ in disguise. He was patron, among many things, of travelers, ferrymen, innkeepers and circus entertainers.
Variations and abbreviations: Jolyon, Jules, Julyan.

Jumoke (pron. J'mókhi)

Origin/meaning: Yoruba 'everyone loves the child'.
A Nigerian name that can be used for both boys and girls.

Justin

Origin/meaning: Latin 'just'.
A name borne by two 5th-century Byzantine Emperors.
Variations and abbreviations: Giustino (It), Giusto, Justinian, Justino (Sp), Justinus, Justus, Yestin (Wel).

K

Kai

Origin/meaning: origin uncertain, possibly from the Roman name Caius, 'rejoice'.
The name may be related to Kay or perhaps have its own roots in Scandinavian languages, in which case its original meaning might be 'hen'.

Kamuzu

Origin/meaning: Nguni 'medicinal'.
This name comes from the South of Africa.
Variation: Kamazu.

Kane

Origin/meaning: Gaelic Irish 'little battle'.
An Anglicized form of an old Irish name.

Boys' Names

Kant
Origin/meaning: Sanskrit 'lover'.
This is found as a name in its own right, and also as a typical masculine suffix to a name ending in a, i or e, e.g. Suryakant.

Kanti (pron. Kantee)
Origin/meaning: Sanskrit 'sun's rays' or 'beauty'.
Found throughout India but less popular than it used to be.

Karl
Origin/meaning: Old German 'man'.
A form of Charles q.v.
Variation: Carl.

Kashyapa
Origin/meaning: unknown.
This is the name of one of the ancient Hindu saints of India.

Kay
Origin/meaning: from the Roman name Gaius or Caius, 'rejoice'.
This is the English spelling of the Welsh name, Cai. Sir Kay was one of the characters from the Tales of King Arthur and his Knights of the Round Table, who was known for his boastfulness.
Variations: Cai (Wel), Caius, Gaius, Kai, Kaye, Key.

Keith
Origin/meaning: Scots Gaelic 'wood'.
This is a Scots last name taken from several Scottish places which have the name. It came into use as a first name in the 19th century when last names became popular as first names.

Kenneth
Origin/meaning: Scots Gaelic 'handsome'.
This is primarily a Scots name although there are native forms in other Celtic areas. Kenneth I (Coinneach) MacAlpine of Scotland was a 9th-century king who kept the Danes out of Scotland. He united his people with the Picts after defeating them in 846, and greatly increased the power of Scotland.
Variations and abbreviations: Canice (Ir), Cennydd (Wel), Ken, Kenny. See also Kevin.

Kentigern
Origin/meaning: Old Welsh 'head chief'.
St Kentigern, d.612, also known by his nickname Mungo, was a Scot who brought Christianity to his native area of Lothian. He is the patron saint of Glasgow and his symbols, a ring and a fish, appear on the city's coat of arms.

" Sometimes the laughter in mothering is the recognition of the ironies and absurdities. Sometimes, though, it's just pure, unthinking delight. "

Barbara Schapiro

Boys' Names

Kevin
Origin/meaning: Old Irish 'handsome at birth'.
This name is similar in meaning to the Scots name Kenneth q.v. St Kevin, d.618, was, according to tradition, a Leinster nobleman who founded a monastery at Glendelough. He is said to have died at the age of 120.
Variations and abbreviations: Kev, Kevan.

Khan
Origin/meaning: Sanskrit 'king', 'lord' or 'ruler'.
Khan added to Muslim names indicates respect as for the Aga Khan. Genghis Khan, 1162–1227, changed his name from Temujin to Genghis Khan which means 'very mighty ruler'.

Kian
Origin/meaning: Irish 'ancient'.
A variant of an old Irish name Cian that has become popular.
Variation: Keane.

Kieran
Origin/meaning: Old Irish 'black-haired'.
This is a diminutive of an Old Irish name Ciar, meaning black or black-haired. The Irish place-name Kerry means the home of Ciar's people or the home of dark-haired people.

Kim
Origin/meaning: Old English 'cyne' – 'royal'. From the last name Kimball 'royal hill' or Kimberley 'royal meadow'.
This name became popular for boys after the publication in 1901 of Rudyard Kipling's book 'Kim'. It has now become equally popular for girls.

Kingsley
Origin/meaning: Old English 'from the king's wood'.
An English last name that came into use as a first name in the 19th century. It may have been given to honor Charles Kingsley, 1819–1875, the popular Victorian novelist, author of 'The Water Babies'.

Kirk
Origin/meaning: Old Norse 'church'.
Kirk is a common last name in the areas of Scotland and the North of England which were invaded by the Vikings. Kirk is now used as a first name.
Variation: Kirke.

Krishna
Origin/meaning: Hindu.
Krishna is regarded by most Hindus as the greatest and most complete incarnation of the god Vishnu. His story is found in many stories and poems, most notably the 9th-century 'Bhagavata Purana'. Krishna was a defender of justice and slew many wrongdoers and evil demons.

Kurt
Origin/meaning: Old German 'bold counselor'.
An alternative spelling of Curt, a short form of Conrad q.v.
Variations and abbreviations: see Conrad.

Kusum-chandra
Origin/meaning: Sanskrit 'flower'.
The equivalent of the feminine Kusum with the addition of the typical male suffix – chandra. The a at the end should not be pronounced or it becomes the female name meaning 'moon'.

Kwame
Origin/meaning: Akan 'born on Saturday'.
Similar names are Kwasi – born on Sunday; Kwakoa – born on Wednesday.

Kyle
Origin/meaning: English 'narrow channel'.
A name that originally came from a Scottish last name and place name, Kyle is now widely used as a first name.

L

Lachlan (pron. Loklan)
Origin/meaning: Scots Gaelic 'from the lake (fiord) land' i.e. 'a Viking'.
This is a Scots first name and last name.

Lance
Origin/meaning: Old German 'land'.
The original French name from which Lancelot (little Lance) developed.
Variations and abbreviations: see Lancelot.

Boys' Names

Lancelot

Origin/meaning: Old German 'land'.

This is a French diminutive of the name Lance and means 'little Lance'. The tale of Lancelot's illicit love for Guinevere, King Arthur's wife, became one of the best known stories of the Arthurian romance.

Variations and abbreviations: Lance, Lancelin, Lancelyn, Lando (Ger), Lanslet, Launce, Launcelot.

Latif

Origin/meaning: Arabic 'pleasant'.

A common Muslim name.

Variation: Lateef (E Africa).

Laurence

Origin/meaning: Latin 'from Laurentium' (the city of laurels).

This name probably became popular because laurel leaves were the victor's traditional crown. It was rare in England before the Norman Conquest. During the Middle Ages its popularity increased and it was usually given to honor St Laurence, a Deacon of Rome. He was martyred in 258 for presenting to the Prefect the city's poor and sick when asked to hand over the church's treasure. In English-speaking countries the spellings Laurence and Lawrence are equally valid.

Variations and abbreviations: Lanty (Ir), Larry, Lars (Swed), Lauren, Laurenz (Ger), Laurens (Dut), Laurent (Fr), Laurentius (Ger/Dut), Laurien, Lauritz (Dan), Lauro (It), Lawrence, Lawrie, Lawry, Lonnie, Lonny, Loren, Lorens, Lorenzo (Ger/Dut), Lorenzo (It), Lorin, Lorrie, Lorry.

Lawrence

Origin/meaning: Latin 'from Laurentium' (the city of laurels).

An alternative English spelling of Laurence q.v. It is the spelling most often used as a last name.

Variations and abbreviations: see Laurence.

Leabua

Origin/meaning: Sotho 'you speak'.

This name is much used in the South of Africa.

Leander

Origin/meaning: Greek 'lion-like'.

A name occasionally used because of the Greek legend of Hero and Leander.

Lee

Origin/meaning: Old English 'meadow'.

An English last name adopted in the 19th century as a first name. Originally a masculine name it is now used equally for girls.

Variations: Lea, Leigh.

Leo

Origin/meaning: Greek/Latin 'lion'.
A pre-Christian name, it was adopted as a Christian name because of the Roman St Leo the Great, 390–461. Also a short form of names beginning with Leo.

Leon

Origin/meaning: Greek 'lion'.
The original Greek form of the Latin word leo.
Variations: Léon (Fr), Léonce (Fr), Leone (It), Leonz (Ger), Lyon.

Leonard

Origin/meaning: Latin, Old German 'lion-bold'.
In the Middle Ages St Leonard was much loved, particularly among Crusaders, who regarded him as the patron saint of prisoners.
Variations and abbreviations: Leander (Ger), Len, Lenard, Lennard, Lennart (Scand), Lennie, Lenny, Leo, Leon, Léonard (Fr), Leonardo (It), Leonerd, Leonhard (Ger), Leinhard (Swiss). See also Leander, Leo, Leon, Lionel, Singh.

Leopold

Origin/meaning: Old German 'people-bold'.
A German name, Leopold was used in 19th-century Britain, because of Queen Victoria's uncle, Leopold I, 1790–1865, King of the Belgians. A sensible moderate man, he was much respected and Queen Victoria named one of her own sons after him.
Variations and abbreviations: Leo, Leobold, Léopold (Fr), Leopoldo (It), Luitpold.

Leroy

Origin/meaning: French 'king'.
This name is common in the US where it may have been taken from the Northern French last name Le Royer, which means 'wheelmaker'. However it is undoubtedly intended to mean 'le roi' – king.

Leslie

Origin/meaning: Scots Gaelic 'garden by the pool'.
The usual spelling of the Scottish last name when used as a masculine name. It came into use as a personal name in the 19th century, helped along by its aristocratic connections, being the last name of the Earls of Rothes.
Variations and abbreviations: Lee, Les, Lesley, Lezlie.

Lester

Origin/meaning: Old English 'Leicester'.
This is an English last name derived from the place-name. It has become well established as a personal name since the 19th century.

L

Boys' Names

Levi
Origin/meaning: Hebrew 'associated' or 'joined'.
An old Biblical name that is more often found in the US than Britain.

Lewis
Origin/meaning: Welsh 'lion-like' or from the name of the Celtic god Luel.
This is an Anglicized form of Lewys, a short form of the Welsh name Llywelyn. It is quite unconnected with the English version of the French Louis.

Liam
Origin/meaning: Old German, English 'determined protector'.
A short version of a Gaelic form of William – Uilliam – that has become extremely popular as a first name, for example the lead singer of the band 'Oasis', Liam Gallagher.

Lindsay
Origin/meaning: Old English. Uncertain, possibly 'Lincoln's island'.
A Scottish aristocratic last name adopted as a male and female first name.
Variations and abbreviations: Lin, Lindsey (Eng), Linsay, Linsey, Lyn, Lynsey.

Linus
Origin/meaning: Latin 'flaxen-haired'.
Possibly a name derived from the Latin word for flax. It is well known because of the Peanuts cartoons in which the character Linus appears.

Lionel
Origin/meaning: Latin/French 'little lion'.
The French diminutive of Leon q.v. it has been used in Britain since the Middle Ages.
Variations: Lionello (It), Lyonel. See also Leo, Leon, Leonard.

Lloyd
Origin/meaning: Welsh 'gray' or 'brown'.
This is a common Welsh last name occasionally used as a first name.
Variation: Floyd.

Llyr
Origin/meaning: Welsh mythology. Llyr was a sea god. He was the father of Branwen. The name Lear, used by Shakespeare for his play 'King Lear', 1607, is thought to be based on it.
Variations: Lear, Leir.

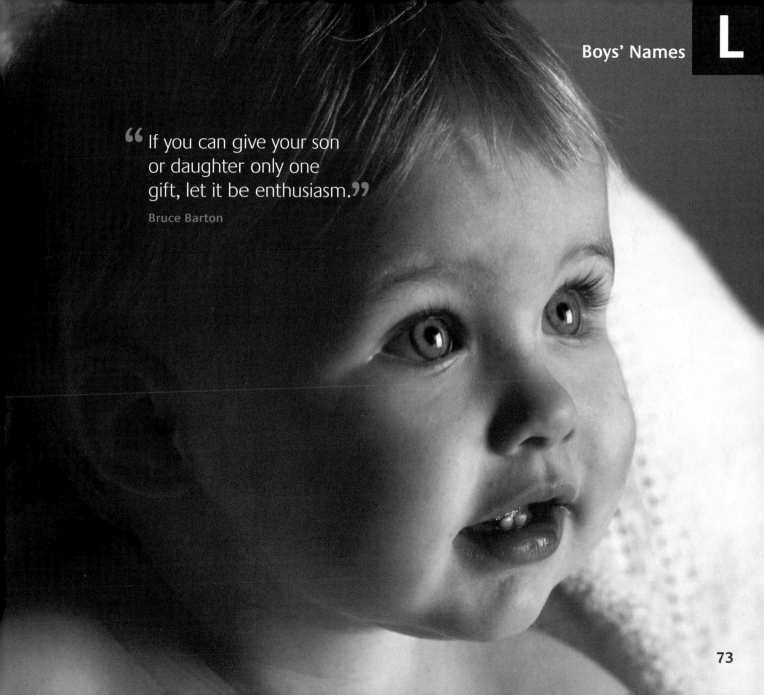

"If you can give your son or daughter only one gift, let it be enthusiasm."

Bruce Barton

Boys' Names

Llywelyn (pron. Chloowellin)
Origin/meaning: uncertain. May be Welsh 'like a lion' or a reference to the Celtic god Luel. This is one of the most popular Welsh names perhaps because it was borne by two famous Welsh princes, Llywelyn ap Iorwerth, d.1240, and his nephew Llywelyn ap Gruffydd, d.1282, the last Welsh Prince of Wales.
Variations and abbreviations: Flewelin, Fluellen, Leoline (Eng), Lewellings, Lewis (Eng), Llelo, Llew, Llewelin, Llowelin, Lyn, Wellings.

Logan
Origin/meaning: Scottish 'little hollow'.
A place name turned last name that is now widely used as a given name.

Louis (pron. Lóuee or Lóuiss)
Origin/meaning: Old German 'glorious battle'.
The original Teutonic form of this name was Chlodovech. Chlodovech, 465–511, was the first Merovingian king of the Western Franks (France). In Latin documents Chlodovech was known either as Clovis or Ludovicus. Ludovicus developed into the French name Louis. It has remained a popular French name for over a thousand years. There have been eighteen French kings who have borne the name.
Variations and abbreviations: Aloys (Provençal), Aloysius, Lew, Lewes, Lewis (Eng), Lodewig (Ger), Lou, Louie, Louis (Fr/Scot), Lovis, Lowes (Med/Eng), Lowis, Lodovico (It), Ludovic (Scot), Ludovico (It), Luigi (It).

Luca
Origin/meaning: Greek 'from Lucania', a region of southern Italy.
This Italian form of Luke is now used in the English-speaking world.

Lucas
Origin/meaning: Greek 'from Lucania'.
This is a Latin form of the name better known in England as Luke. In France and Germany Lucas is a common form of Luke.
Variations and abbreviations: see Luke.

Lucian (pron. Lóosean or Lóoshan)
Origin/meaning: Latin 'light'.
St Lucian, d.312, was a theologian from Antioch who revised the Greek version of the Old Testament and the gospels.
Variation: Lucien (Fr).

Lucius
Origin/meaning: Latin 'light'.
This name was a pre-Christian Roman name, probably used for a child born at first light of day. The English feminine form Lucy is very popular.
Variations: Lucian, Luciano (It), Lucien (Fr), Lucillio (It), Lucio (It), Luzian, Luzius (Ger).

Ludovic

Origin/meaning: Old German 'glorious battle'. This is a variation of the name Lewis q.v. through one of its Latin forms, Ludovicus.
Variations and abbreviations: Lodowick (Eng), Lodovico (It), Ludo, Ludovico (It), Ludwig (Ger). See also Lewis.

Luke

Origin/meaning: Greek 'from Lucania'. Sometimes given as 'wolf'.
This is the name of one of the four Evangelists, and author of the Acts of the Apostles. He was a Greek and a doctor, called by St Paul 'our beloved Luke, the physician'. He is the patron saint of doctors.
Variations and abbreviations: Loukas (Gr), Luc (Fr), Luca (It), Lucano (It), Lucas (Fr/Eng/Ger), Lucio (Sp), Luck (Eng), Lukas (Ger/Scand).

Lyall

Origin/meaning: French 'from Lyons' ('the hillfort') or French 'little lion'.
An English last name not infrequently used as a first name.

Lyn

Origin/meaning: uncertain. Possibly Welsh 'like a lion' or a reference to the Celtic god Luel.
A Welsh male name. A short form of Llewelyn q.v. now used as an independent name.

Lyndon

Origin/meaning: Old English 'from the lime tree hill'.
An English place-name which became a last name.
Variation: Lindon.

M

Madhukar (pron. Madtookarr)

Origin/meaning: Sanskrit 'bee'.
The masculine equivalent of Madhuri q.v.

Magnus

Origin/meaning: Latin 'great'.
This adjective became a name in its own right.
Variation: Manus (Ir).

Boys' Names

Malcolm
Origin/meaning: Old Scots 'servant of Columba'.
A popular Scottish name for hundreds of years because of the influence of St Columba who brought Christianity to a large part of Scotland.
Abbreviation: Mal.

Malik
Origin/meaning: Arabic 'the king'.
A popular Muslim name.

Manfred
Origin/meaning: Old German 'man-peace'.
A pre-Conquest name adopted by the Normans and introduced by them into England. Byron wrote a drama 'Manfred', 1819.
Variations: Manfredo (It), Manfried (Ger).

Marcel
Origin/meaning: Latin 'little Marcus' from 'Mars' (the Roman god of war) i.e. 'warlike'.
The French form of the Latin Marcellus, a diminutive of Marcus.
Variations: Marcello (It), Marcellus, Marzellus (Ger). See also Mark.

Marcus
Origin/meaning: Latin 'of Mars' (the Roman god of war), i.e. 'warlike'.
This is the Roman name which developed into the Christian name Mark q.v.
Variations and abbreviations: see Mark.

Marius
Origin/meaning: Latin, from the name of the Roman Marius family, probably connected with Mars, god of war.
This name was one of many classical names re-introduced during the 16th-century renaissance period.
Variation: Mario (It). See also Marcus, Mark, Martin.

Mark
Origin/meaning: Latin 'of Mars' (the Roman god of war), i.e. 'warlike'.
This name comes from the popular Roman name Marcus. It became an established Christian name because of St Mark who wrote one of the four gospels. St Mark is closely associated with the city of Venice for in 829, his body was brought there after his martyrdom.
Variations: Marek (Slav), Marc (Fr), Marcel (Fr), Marco (It), Marcos (Sp), Marcus, Marko, Markus (Ger/Dut/Scand), Marks, Marx.

Marlon
Origin/meaning: origin unknown, possibly Old French 'little Mark'.
A name whose original popularity was due almost entirely to the great actor Marlon Brando.

Martin
Origin/meaning: Latin 'of Mars' (the Roman god of war), i.e. 'warlike'.
This was a popular name in the Middle Ages when it was given to honor St Martin of Tours, 315–397. A young Roman officer, he gave half his cloak to a poor beggar whom he later recognized as Christ.
Variations and abbreviations: Mart, Martainn (Scot), Marten, Martie, Martinet (Fr), Martino (It/Sp), Marton, Marty, Martyn, Merten, Morten (Dan). See also Marcus, Mark.

Mason
Origin/meaning: English 'mason'.
An occupational last name that is now used as a given name.

Masud
Origin/meaning: Arabic 'fortunate'.
This is a common Muslim name found in all Muslim countries.
Variations and abbreviations: Mansur, Masood, Massur.

Matsimela
Origin/meaning: Sotho 'roots'.
This name comes from the African state of Lesotho, formerly known as Basutoland, in South Africa.

Matthew
Origin/meaning: Hebrew 'gift of Jehovah'.
In England the name developed from Mattheu, which was introduced by the Normans. It was given to honor St Matthew, the Apostle and Evangelist.
Variations and abbreviations: Mat, Mateo (Port/Sp), Mathias, Matias, Matt, Matteo (It), Matthaeus, Matthäus (Swiss), Mattheus, Matthias (Ger), Matthieu (Fr), Mattias, Mattie, Matty.

Maurice
Origin/meaning: Latin 'a man from Mauretania' (Morocco).
This Roman name was introduced as a Christian name because of the 3rd-century St Maurice (Mauritius). He was said to have been the commanding officer of a legion of Christian Roman soldiers who refused to obey orders to take part in heathen rituals. The English form of Mauritius was based on the more general Latin adjective Maurus – a Moor. In the 19th and 20th centuries Maurice has become the accepted first name form. English folk dances based on characters from the tales of Robin Hood became known as Morris (Moorish) dances.
Variations and abbreviations: Maur (Fr/Ger), Mauricio (Port/Sp), Maurie, Maurise, Mauritius (Ger), Maurits (Dut), Mauriz, Maurizio (It), Mauro (It), Maurus (Ger), Maury, Morie, Moritz (Swiss), Moriz, Morris, Morry.

Boys' Names

Mawulawde (pron. Mahwoolawaydáy)
Origin/meaning: Ewe 'God will provide'.
This name comes from Ghana in West Africa.

Mawuli (pron. Máhwoolee)
Origin/meaning: Ewe 'there is a God'.
A popular name in Ghana.

Max
Origin/meaning: Latin 'greatest'.
A short form of Maximilian or Maxwell. It has become popular since the end of the19th century as an independent name.
Variations and abbreviations: see Maximilian.

Maximilian
Origin/meaning: Latin 'greatest'.
This is derived from the Latin word maximus. The name became popular in Germany because of the highly successful and popular Emperor Maximilian I, 1459–1519.
Variations and abbreviations: Mac, Massimiliano (It), Massimo (It), Max, Maxime (Fr), Maximilien (Fr), Maximus.

Maxwell
Origin/meaning: Scots/Old English 'Magnus's well'.
This is a Scottish place-name which became a last name. It has been used consistently since the 19th century as a first name.
Variations and abbreviations: Mac, Max.

Mayur
Origin/meaning: Sanskrit 'peacock'.
One of Shiv's sons, Kumara or Skanda, the six-headed god of war, is usually depicted riding on a peacock.

Melvin
Origin/meaning: French/English 'town on a hill' or Old English 'sword friend'.
This is an English last name which has been established since the 19th century as a personal name.
Variations and abbreviations: Mel, Melville, Melvyn.

Merlin
Origin/meaning: Old Welsh 'sea hill'.
This name is still used occasionally in Wales. It is widely known as the name of King Arthur's magician. Tales of Merlin can be found in all the sources of the Arthurian Romance.
Variation: Merlyn.

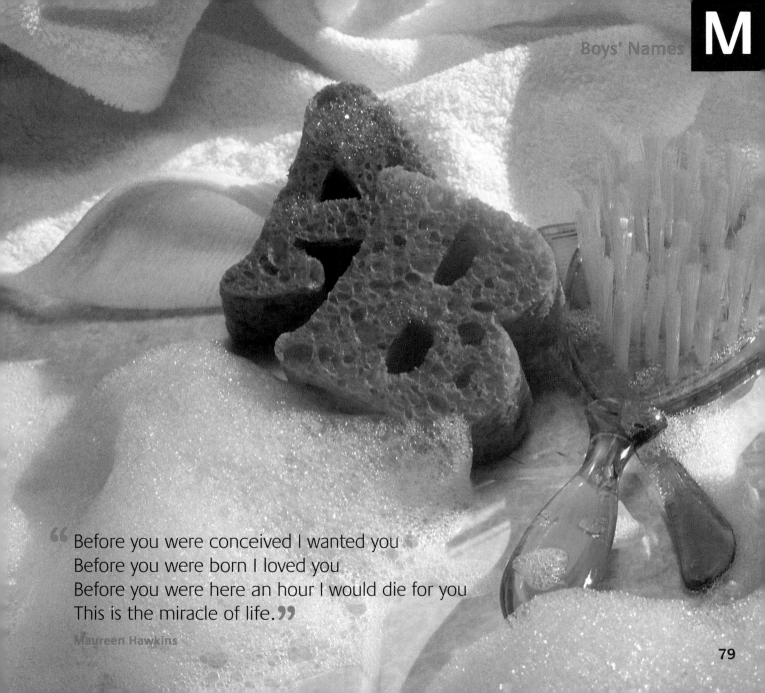

"Before you were conceived I wanted you
Before you were born I loved you
Before you were here an hour I would die for you
This is the miracle of life."

Maureen Hawkins

Boys' Names

Mervyn
Origin/meaning: Old English 'famous friend' or Celtic 'fair sea'.
This last name has English and Welsh forms and the two may be quite separate. Used as a first name since the 19th century.
Variations and abbreviations: Merfyn (Wel), Merv, Mervin. See also Morgan, Murdoch, Murray.

Michael
Origin/meaning: Hebrew 'Who is like the Lord?'
Michael is the name of the archangel who led the angels into battle to cast out Satan. Like St George he is usually represented slaying a dragon. Not surprisingly, St Michael was the patron saint of soldiers.
Variations and abbreviations: Meikle, Micah, Michal, Michel (Fr), Michele (It), Mick, Mickey, Mickie, Micky, Miguel (Sp/Port), Mikael (Scand), Mike, Mikel, Mikey, Mikhail (Russ), Mikkel (Dan), Mischa (Russ), Mitch, Mitchell.

Mihir
Background: Sanskrit 'sun'.
A popular Indian name.

Miles
Origin/meaning: Old German. Uncertain, possibly 'merciful' or Latin 'soldierly'.
A popular medieval name, which was successfully revived in the 19th century and is still in use today.
Variations and abbreviations: Milo (Ger/Ir), Myles.

Milo
Origin/meaning: origin uncertain, possibly Latin 'soldierly'.
This variation of Miles has become increasingly widespread in its own right.

Mitchell
Origin/meaning: Hebrew 'Who is like God?'
A last name that came from Michael and that is now used as a first name.
Variation and abbreviation: Mitch.

Mohammed
Origin/meaning: Arabic/Swahili 'praised'.
Mohammed is a religious title that prefixes the personal name.
Mohammed, the Prophet, died in AD 632 having created a new faith called Islam. His teachings are found in the Koran.
Variations: Mehemmet, Muhammed.

Mohan
Origin/meaning: a Hindu name for Krishna q.v.
This was Gandhi's first name, used with the addition of the typical male suffix -das, i.e. Mohandas Gandhi.

Morgan

Origin/meaning: Old Welsh 'sea bright'.

Morgan was a 7th-century Welsh prince who gave his name to the area of South Wales known as Glamorgan.

Variation: Morgen.

Moses

Origin/meaning: Egyptian 'saved from the water', Hebrew 'law-giver'.

Moses was chosen by God to lead the Israelites out of slavery in Egypt to the Promised Land (see the 2nd Book of Moses – Exodus).

Variations and abbreviations: Moshe (Hebrew), Moss, Moyse, Mozes.

Moyo (pron. Móyo)

Origin/meaning: Ngoni 'good health'.

This name comes from the Central African state of Malawi.

Mungo

Origin/meaning: Gaelic 'lovable', 'most dear'.

This was an adjective used to describe St Kentigern, d.612. It came to be used as an alternative name for him and then as a first name.

Variation: Munghu.

Murdoch

Origin/meaning: Scots Gaelic 'man of the sea'.

A Scots first name that developed as a last name and is now used as a first name again.

Variation: Murtagh (Ir).

Murray

Origin/meaning: Scots Gaelic 'sea settlement'.

This is a Scottish place-name (Moray is a Scots county) which became a last name. In the 19th century it was adopted as a first name, helped by the fact that it is the last name of the Dukes of Atholl and of the Earls of Moray.

Variation: Moray. See also Murdoch, Morgan, Mervyn.

Mwai (pron. M'wáhee)

Origin/meaning: Ngoni 'good fortune'.

A name from the Central African state of Malawi.

N

Nasim
Origin/meaning: Arabic 'discipliner'.
A Muslim name.
Variation: Nizam.

Nassor
Origin/meaning: Swahili 'victorious'.
A name found in Tanzania in East Africa.
See also Victor.

Nathan
Origin/meaning: Hebrew 'gift'.
This is the name of an Old Testament prophet. It is also used as a short form of Nathaniel q.v.
Variation and abbreviation: Nat.

Nathaniel
Origin/meaning: Hebrew 'God has given'.
This is the first name of the Apostle who is better known by his family name, Bartholomew.
Variations and abbreviations: Nat, Nataniel (Sp), Nataniele (It), Nathan, Nathanael, Nathaneal, Natty. See also Theodore and Jonathan.

Nazir
Origin/meaning: Arabic 'victorious'.
This is a Muslim name.
Variations: Nasser, Nassor (E Africa), Nasr.

Neal(e)
Origin/meaning: Old Irish 'champion'.
This is one of the many spellings of the name Neil, which is a form of Niall (Irish) and Nigel q.v. It usually appears as a surname.
Variations and abbreviations: see Nigel.

Neil (pron. Neeal)
Origin/meaning: Old Irish 'champion'.
This is a form of the Irish name Niall, which developed from the word 'niadh' and is the direct equivalent of Nigel q.v.
Variations and abbreviations: see Nigel.

Neville

Origin/meaning: French 'new city' (Neuville is a place in Normandy.)

This is a Norman French last name which came over to England at the time of the Conquest in the form of de Nevil. The Nevilles were an important aristocratic family in the Middle Ages. It was therefore an almost inevitable addition to the number of aristocratic last names (Sidney, Percy, Russell, Ashley etc.) which came into use in the 19th century.

Variations: Nevel, Nevil, Nevill.

Niall (pron. Nýe-all)

Origin/meaning: Old Irish 'champion'.

A modern Irish name, the equivalent of the English Nigel. Both names stem from the Old Irish 'niadh' meaning champion. The form Neil is also common in Ireland.

Variations and abbreviations: see Nigel.

Nicholas

Origin/meaning: Greek 'victory of the people'.

This pre-Christian Greek name was adopted as a Christian name because of the veneration for St Nicholas, a 4th-century bishop of Myra in Asia Minor. Initially popular in the Eastern church (the name is still much used in Eastern Europe) his fame spread to Western Europe in the early Middle Ages.

Variations and abbreviations: Claus (Ger), Cole, Colet, Colin, Klaas (Dut), Klaus (Ger), Niccolo (It), Nick, Nickie, Nicko, Nicky, Nicol (Med Eng), Nicolas (Fr), Nikita (Russ), Niklaus (Ger), Nikolai (Russ), Nikolaus (Ger).

Nicol

Origin/meaning: Greek 'victory of the people'.

This is one of the earliest English forms of Nicholas. It was used for boys and girls. Itself a common Scottish last name it gave rise to many others, most notably Nicolson.

Variations and abbreviations: see Nicholas.

Nigel

Origin/meaning: Old Irish 'champion'.

This name developed from the Irish Celtic 'niadh' meaning champion.

Variations and abbreviations: Neal, Neale, Neel, Nele, Neil, Neill, Neils (Scand), Nels (Scand), Nial, Niall, Niel, Niels (Scand), Nils (Scand).

Ninian

Origin/meaning: uncertain, possibly a Celtic corruption of the Latin 'vivianus' (Vivian) – 'full of life'.

This was the name of an early British missionary, St Ninian, d.432, who converted the Southern Picts of Scotland to Christianity.

Variations: Ninias, Ninnidh (Ir), Nynia.

Boys' Names

Nkrumah
Origin/meaning: Akan 'ninth born'.
This is a Ghanaian name.

Noël
Origin/meaning: Latin/Old French 'birth day', i.e. 'Christmas'.
This French word for Christmas has been used as a name for children born at the Christmas season since the early Middle Ages.
Variations: Natale (It), Noel, Nowel (Eng), Nowell.

Norman
Origin/meaning: Old English/Old German 'north man'.
This is a pre-Conquest name. It developed in England to describe the many invaders from Scandinavia, to the North of the British Isles, who repeatedly invaded the country after the departure of the Romans.
Variations and abbreviations: Norm, Normand, Normann (Ger).

Norris
Origin/meaning: Old French 'northerner'.
This is a family name occasionally used as a first name.

Nural
Origin/meaning: Arabic 'born in daylight'.
A popular Arabic name.
Variation: Nuru (E African).

Oberon
Origin/meaning: Old German 'little elf-ruler'.
An alternative spelling of Auberon q.v. which was used by Shakespeare as an appropriate name for the king of the fairies in 'A Midsummer Night's Dream'.

Octavius
Origin/meaning: Latin 'eighth'.
A name given to an eighth son or child. Octavius was the brother-in-law of Julius Caesar. His son, Octavianus, became the Emperor Augustus.

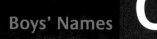

"It is not until you become a mother
that your judgment slowly turns to
compassion and understanding."

Erma Bombeck

Boys' Names

Odysseus
Origin/meaning: uncertain. Possibly Etruscan 'wanderer' – sometimes given as 'hater'.
The original Greek version of Ulysses q.v.

Okechuku (pron. Okehchóoku)
Origin/meaning: Yoruba 'God's gift'.
A Nigerian name.

Okpara (pron. Okpára)
Origin/meaning: Ibo 'first son'.
This name comes from Nigeria.

Olaf
Origin/meaning: Old Norse 'ancestor-inheritance/remains'.
The Danes who invaded Britain brought the name with them but it died out after the Norman Conquest. It probably survives as the English Oliver q.v. and French Olivier.

Oliver
Origin/meaning: uncertain. Possibly Old Norse 'ancestor-inheritance/remains', from Anleifr. Sometimes given as 'olive tree'.
The name is likely to have the Old Norse meaning of the Scandinavian name Olaf q.v. Oliver was the form used in England in the Middle Ages.
Variations and abbreviations: Noll (Med Eng), Nolly, Olaf (Scand), Olav (Scand), Oliverio (Sp), Olivier (Fr), Oliviero (It), Ollie, Olly.

Olu
Origin/meaning: Yoruba 'pre-eminent'.
This name comes from Nigeria.

Omar
Origin/meaning: Arab (and Swahili) 'highest'.
Omar, 581–644, was the second Khalif. He was the father of one of Mohammed's nine wives. His military skill extended his empire across North Africa, Persia and Syria.
Variations: Omari (Swahili), Umar.

Orlando
Origin/meaning: Old German 'fame-land' usually given as 'famous man of the land'.
This is the Italian form of the English Rowland and French Roland q.v. It was found in England during the Renaissance period and Shakespeare used it in his play 'As You Like It'.

Orson

Origin/meaning: Latin 'bear'.
This is the English form of the Italian name Orso.

Orville

Origin/meaning: Old French 'golden town'.
A rare name familiar because of the US aviation pioneer Orville Wright, 1871–1948.

Osakwe (pron. Osárkway)

Origin/meaning: Benin 'God agrees'.
A Nigerian name. The word Os – God, appears in many Nigerian names, for example Osahar – 'God hears', Osayaba – 'God forgives' and Osaze – 'liked by God'.

Osbert

Origin/meaning: Old English 'god-famous'.
One of several Old English names e.g. Oscar, Osborn, which contain the word Os, meaning God. It was found in Northumbria where Viking influence was strong and it has a very similar Old Norse equivalent.

Osborn

Origin/meaning: Old English 'god-warrior' or Old Norse 'god-bear'.
A pre-Conquest name which developed primarily as a last name in the Middle Ages, now found as a personal name again.
Variations and abbreviations: Osborne, Osbourne, Ossy.

Oscar

Origin/meaning: Old Norse 'god spear', i.e. 'divine spear'.
A Scandinavian name which was introduced into Britain by the Viking invaders, although the Anglo-Saxon equivalent may well have existed.
Variations and abbreviations: Asger (Dan), Ansgar, Osgar (Ir), Oskar (Ger/Scand), Ossie, Ossy, Ozzie, Ozzy.

Osgar

Origin/meaning: Old Norse 'sea-spear', i.e. 'divine spear'.
The Irish form of Oscar q.v.

Osmond

Origin/meaning: Old English/Old Norse 'god-protection', i.e. 'divine protection'.
Like Osbert, Oswald and Oscar, this name developed in several countries simultaneously. It survived the Conquest because the Normans had already adopted it.
Variations and abbreviations: Osmonde, Osmund, Ozzy.

Boys' Names

Oswald
Origin/meaning: Old English 'god-power'.
Another Old English Northumbrian name, like Osbert q.v., which is very similar to an Old Norse name.
Variations and abbreviations: Ossy, Oswell, Ozzy, Waldo.

Otto
Origin/meaning: Old German 'of the fatherland' or 'rich'.
The version of the Old German name Odo which has survived most successfully into the 20th century.
Variations and abbreviations: Odo, Oddo, Odilo, Othello, Otho.

Owen
Origin/meaning: uncertain. Possibly Old Scots/Irish 'young warrior' or Welsh 'lamb' or Old Welsh 'well born'.
One of the most common Welsh names both as a first name and as a last name.
Variations: Eugene, Ewen (Scot), Owain (Wel), Ywain (Old Wel).

P

Paddy
Origin/meaning: Latin 'patrician'.
An Irish familiar form of Patrick q.v. and occasionally of the feminine form Patricia. It developed from the Irish version of the name, Pádraig.
Variation: Patty

Pádraig (pron. Pórreg)
Origin/meaning: Latin 'patrician'.
The native Irish form of Patrick q.v.
Variation: Pádraic.

Paris
Origin/meaning: Greek/English, legendary character of Troy.
Paris was the son of Priam and the man who fell in love with the already-married Helen. His determination to have her as his wife provoked the Trojan War. Sometimes used as a name for girls.

Parker
Origin/meaning: English 'park keeper'.
Originally an occupation name, and still more usual as a last name, Parker is also now found as a given name.

Patrick

Origin/meaning: Latin 'patrician' i.e. aristocratic.

This is a name long associated with Ireland and to a lesser extent Scotland. St Patrick is, of course, the patron saint of Ireland.

Variations and abbreviations: Paddie, Paddy, Pádraic, Pádraig, Padrig (Wel), Pat, Patric, Patrice (Fr), Patrizio (It), Patrizius (Ger/Dut), Patsy, Patty.

Paul

Origin/meaning: Latin 'small'.

Just as Timothy and Euphemia were long-established Greek personal names adopted as Christian names because they appear in the Bible, so Paul (Paullus) was an established Roman name. Its use as a first name is due to St Paul, who changed his name from the Jewish Saul, after his conversion to Christianity on the road to Damascus.

Variations: Paavo (Finn), Pablo (Sp), Paolo (It), Paolino (It), Paulinus, Paulus, Pavel (Russ), Poul (Dan).

Perceval

Origin/meaning: French 'from Percheval' a village in Normandy.

This is a Norman French last name occasionally used as a first name in England and France since the Middle Ages. The short form Percy soon became a separate last name in its own right.

Variations and abbreviations: Perce, Percival, Percy.

Peregrine

Origin/meaning: Latin 'foreigner', 'traveler', 'pilgrim'.

A rare name, it has been used since the early Middle Ages to honor St Peregrinus, the patron saint of Modena.

Variations and abbreviations: Pellegrino (It), Peregrin (Ger), Perry.

Peter

Origin/meaning: Greek 'stone'.

In John I, v.42, Jesus renamed Simon saying, 'Thou art Simon, the son of Jona: thou shalt be called Cephas, which is by interpretation, a stone'. Since the gospel was written in Greek and the Greek word for stone is petros, Simon came to be known as Simon Peter and later as St Peter.

Variations and abbreviations: Pär (Swed), Parry, Peadar (Ir), Pearce, Peder, Pedro (Sp), Peer (Norway), Per (Swed), Perkin (Med Eng), Perry, Pete, Pierce, Pierre (Fr), Pieter (Dut), Piero (It), Pietro (It), Pyotr (Russ), Pyrs (Wel).

Phelim

Origin/meaning: Old Irish 'ever good'.

A popular Irish name. Sometimes 'translated' to Felix by English speakers.

Variations: Feiolim (Celt), Felim, Felimy.

Boys' Names

Philip

Origin/meaning: Greek 'lover of horses'.

This is the name of one of the Apostles and was therefore much used in the Middle Ages when saints' names were popular.

Variations and abbreviations: Felipe (Sp), Filip (Scand), Filippo (It), Lippo (It), Phil, Philipp (Ger), Philippe (Fr), Philippus (Ger/Dut), Pip.

Phineas

Origin/meaning: uncertain. Sometimes given as Hebrew 'oracle' or Egyptian 'negro'.

This is a Biblical name adopted by 17th-century Puritans, especially in New England. It has always been rare.

Variation: Phinehas.

Piers

Origin/meaning: Greek 'stone'.

The form of Peter q.v. introduced into Britain by the Normans in 1066. It was eventually ousted by the form Peter, which is nearer to the original Greek.

Variations and abbreviations: see Peter.

Placido (pron. Plassido)

Origin/meaning: Latin 'calm'.

An adjective occasionally used as a name, made famous by the great Spanish singer Placido Domingo.

Purushotam (pron. Pooróosotam)

Origin/meaning: Sanskrit 'best of men'.

The name of a Hindu god. Found throughout India.

Quentin

Origin/meaning: Latin 'fifth'.

Quintus was a Roman forename and also the name of a famous tribe, the Quintii, renowned for their exemplary behavior. Two early Roman martyrs, SS Quintino and Quinto, made the name familiar and their names became altered to Quentine in France before it came to England.

Variations and abbreviations: Quinn, Quint, Quintilio (It), Quintin, Quinto (It), Quinton, Quntus (Ger).

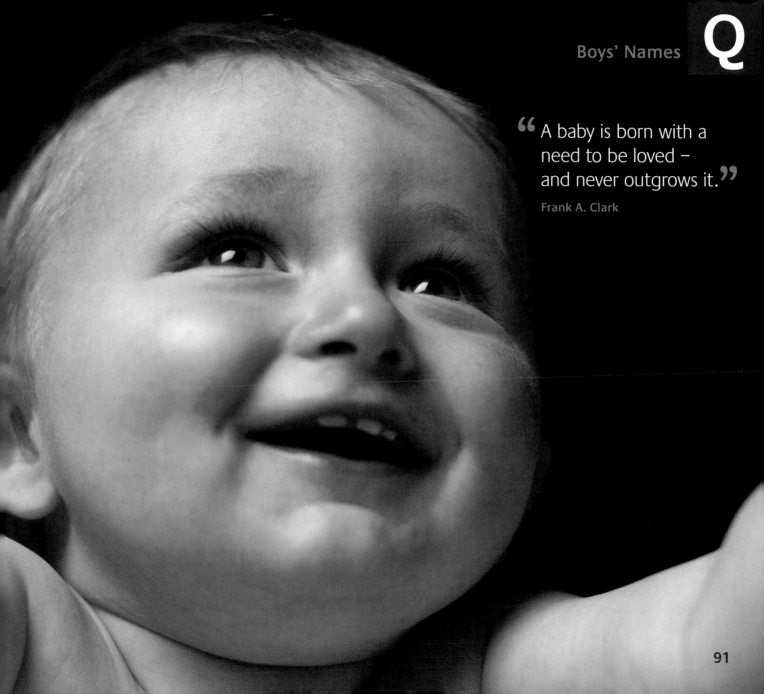

"A baby is born with a
need to be loved –
and never outgrows it."

Frank A. Clark

Boys' Names

Quincy
Origin/meaning: Latin/Old French 'from the fifth place', 'from the fifth son's estate'.
There are several places called Quincy in France and settlers in England at the time of the Conquest brought the name with them. It is most usual as a last name, sometimes with the aristocratic prefix de. Thomas De Quincy, 1785–1859, author of 'Confessions of an English Opium Eater', is an example.
Variations and abbreviations: Quin, Quincey, Quinn.

Quinn
Origin/meaning: Old Irish 'counsel' or (sometimes) Latin 'fifth'.
A common Irish last name used as a first name. It is sometimes found as a short form of Quintin or Quincy.
Variation: Quin.

Quintin
Origin/meaning: Latin 'fifth'.
An alternative spelling of Quentin q.v.

R

Rafe
Origin/meaning: Old Norse/Old English 'wolf counsel'.
A variation of Ralph q.v. which is spelt according to the pronunciation.

Rajan
Origin/meaning: Sanskrit 'king'.
This is the Gujerati version of the name. The Sikh version uses the typical Sikh addition Singh, which means 'lion'.
Variation: Rajinder, Singh (Sikh).

Raksha
Origin/meaning: Sanskrit 'protected'.
This is the name of a Hindu festival (usually in August) when brothers are reminded of their duty to protect their sisters.

Ralph (pron. Rafe. Modern pron. Ralph)
Origin/meaning: Old Norse/Old English 'wolf counsel'.
This (sometimes in the form Radulf) was a pre-Conquest English name. It was also popular with the Normans so it did not die out in England after the Norman Conquest.
Variations and abbreviations: Rafe, Ralf, Raoul (Fr).

Ranald

Origin/meaning: Old German/Old English 'power-might'.
An uncommon spelling of Ronald, the Scottish equivalent of Reynold and its variation Reginald. Unlike Ronald, Ranald has remained distinctively Scottish.

Randal

Origin/meaning: Old English 'shield wolf'.
One of two medieval forms of this pre-Conquest name, the other being Ranulf. Randal has survived into the 20th century as well as giving rise to several last names, including Randle, Ransom, Rankin etc.
Variations and abbreviations: Rand, Randall, Randell, Randolf, Randolph, Randy, Ranulf, Ranulph. See also Ralph.

Randolph

Origin/meaning: Old English 'shield wolf'.
The 18th-century 'classical' version of the old name Ranulf, more commonly found today in the medieval form Randal q.v.

Raphael

Origin/meaning: Hebrew 'God has healed'.
One of the three named archangels in the Bible, together with Gabriel and Michael.
Variations and abbreviations: Rafael, Raffaele (It), Raffaello (It), Raphael (Fr), Rafe, Ray.

Ravi

Origin/meaning: Sanskrit 'sun'.

Ravindra (pron. Ravindr)

Origin/meaning: Sanskrit 'sun-king of heaven'.
Variations: Rabindra, Ravinder Singh (Sikh).

Raymond

Origin/meaning: Old German 'strength protection' or 'counsel protection', i.e. 'strong' or 'wise protector'.
A name found in Britain since it was introduced by the Normans in 1066. It is found in various forms throughout Europe and is also a last name.
Variations and abbreviations: Raimondo (It), Raimund (Ger), Raimundo (Sp), Ramón (Sp), Ray, Raymund, Reamonn (Ir), Reimund (Ger).

Reginald

Origin/meaning: Old German/Old English 'power-might'. Sometimes given as 'powerful judgment'.
This is a late medieval version of the name Reynold from the form which appeared in Latin manuscripts 'Reginaldus'.
Variations and abbreviations: Reg, Reggie, Reginaldo (It), Reginauld (Fr), Rex, Reynold.

Boys' Names

Reuben

Origin/meaning: uncertain. Sometimes given as 'behold, a son'. Possibly Hebrew 'renewer'.
This is a Biblical name. Reuben was one of the sons of Jacob and gave his name to one of the tribes of Israel.
Variations and abbreviations: Rube, Rubén (Sp), Rubin.

Rex

Origin/meaning: Latin 'king'.
A name which appears in the early years of the 20th century presumably to honor the accession of a king (Edward VII) after the long reign of Queen Victoria.

Rhys (pron. Rees)

Origin/meaning: Welsh 'fiery'.
An old name that has become popular in recent times.
Variations: Reece, Rees.

Richard

Origin/meaning: Old English 'rule hard', i.e. 'strong king'.
An Anglo-Saxon name, used by a Kentish king who went as a monk to Europe. The name became established in Europe where there was a similar Old German name and was introduced back into England at the Norman Conquest.
Variations and abbreviations: Diccon (Med Eng), Dick, Dickie, Dicky, Reichard (Ger), Ric, Ricard, Ricardo (Sp), Riccardo (It), Rich, Richardt (Ger), Richart (Dut), Richie, Richy, Rik, Riocard (Ir), Ritchie.

Ridley

Origin/meaning: English 'clearing in the reeds'.
This old place name and last name is best known as the given name of celebrated Hollywood film director Ridley Scott.

Riley

Origin/meaning: English 'clearing in the rye'.
An old place name that is sometimes found as a given name.

Rob

A popular short form of Robert and Robin q.v.

Robert

Origin/meaning: Old German 'fame-bright'.
This name, originally Hrodebert, was the name of a Saxon bishop of the 8th century. His fame made the name popular throughout the Holy Roman Empire.
Variations and abbreviations: Bert, Bertie, Bob, Bobbie, Bobby, Rab, Rabbie, Riobard (Ir), Rob, Robbie, Robby, Roberto (It), Robin, Robrecht (Ger), Rupert.

Robin

Origin/meaning: Old German 'fame-bright'.
An originally French diminutive of Robert. The ending implies affection.

Rocco

Origin/meaning: Old German 'rest'.
This Italian name, equivalent of the English Rock, has become especially popular after pop star Madonna and Guy Ritchie used this name for their son.

Rock

Origin/meaning: Old German 'crow'/'jay' or Old English 'rock'.
A short form of several obsolete names beginning with Roch, such as Rochbert. St Roch or Rock was a 14th-century Frenchman who nursed plague victims while on a pilgrimage to Rome. In the US the name Rock or Rocky is usually an English spelling of the name Rocco, the Italian form of Roch. It is generally used for boys of Italian descent.
Variations and abbreviations: Rocco (It), Roch (Fr), Rochus (Ger/Dut), Rocky.

Roderick

Origin/meaning: Old German 'fame ruler'. Usually given as 'famous ruler'.
One of the most lasting and widespread of the Old German names, Roderick is found in various forms throughout Europe.
Variations and abbreviations: Rod, Rodd, Roddie, Roddy, Roderich (Ger), Roderigo, Rodrigo (Sp/It/Port), Rodrigue (Fr), Rory, Rurik (Scand/Russ), Ruy (Sp).

Roger

Origin/meaning: Old English/Old German 'fame spear'. Usually given as 'famous spearman'.
This ancient name is found in its original form – Hrothgar – in 'Beowulf', the Old English epic poem. The name has been found in its present form since the Middle Ages.
Variations and abbreviations: Rodge, Rodger, Rog, Rogerio (Sp), Rüdiger (Ger), Ruggiero (It), Rutger (Dut), Ruttger.

Roland

Origin/meaning: Old German 'fame land', usually given as 'famous man of the land'.
This is the French version of the name which was brought to England by the Normans in 1066.

Roman

Origin/meaning: Latin, Russian 'Roman'.
This name remains very popular in parts of Eastern Europe and Russia.

Romeo

Origin/meaning: Latin, Italian 'pilgrim to Rome'.

Boys' Names

The name was made famous by Shakespeare in 'Romeo and Juliet'. Its modern resurgence in Britain is more due to England soccer star David Beckham and his wife Victoria naming their second son Romeo.
Variation: Romeus.

Ronald
Origin/meaning: Old German/Old English 'power-might'.
Like the English Reginald q.v. this Scottish name is a development of Reynold.
Variations and abbreviations: Ranald, Reginald, Reynold, Ron, Ronnie.

Rory
Origin/meaning: Gaelic 'red-haired' or Old German 'famous ruler'.
The original Celtic name Ruaridh (Scots) and Rhuadhri (Irish) became Roderigh or, more familiar, Rory.
Variations and abbreviations: Rorie, Roderick, Roger, Roy.

Ross
Origin/meaning: Old Scots 'of the promontory' or Old German 'fame'.
A common Scots last name which has gained popularity in the 20th century as a first name.

Rowan
Origin/meaning: Old Norse 'rowan tree'.
A last name used as a first name, perhaps influenced by the similarity to Rowland.

Rowland
Origin/meaning: Old German 'fame-land', usually given as 'famous man of the land'. This spelling was the most usual in England from the late Middle Ages until the 18th century. In the 19th century the fashion for medieval culture led to a preference for the version brought to England by the Normans – Roland q.v.
Variations and abbreviations: Orlando (It), Roland (Fr/Ger), Rolando (It/Port/Sp), Roldan (Sp), Rolland, Rollo, Rolly, Rowley, Rowly, Ruland (Ger).

Roy
Origin/meaning: Celtic 'red', 'red-haired'.
Sometimes thought to be the equivalent of the Spanish Ruy – ruler, through the French word roi – king.
Variations: Rory (Scot/Ir), Ruffino (It), Rufus.

Rudolph
Origin/meaning: Old German 'fame-wolf'.
A modern German form of a pre-Conquest name.
Variations and abbreviations: Rodolf, Rodolphe (Fr), Rolph, Rodolf, Rodolfo (It), Rodolphe (Fr), Rudolf, Rudy.

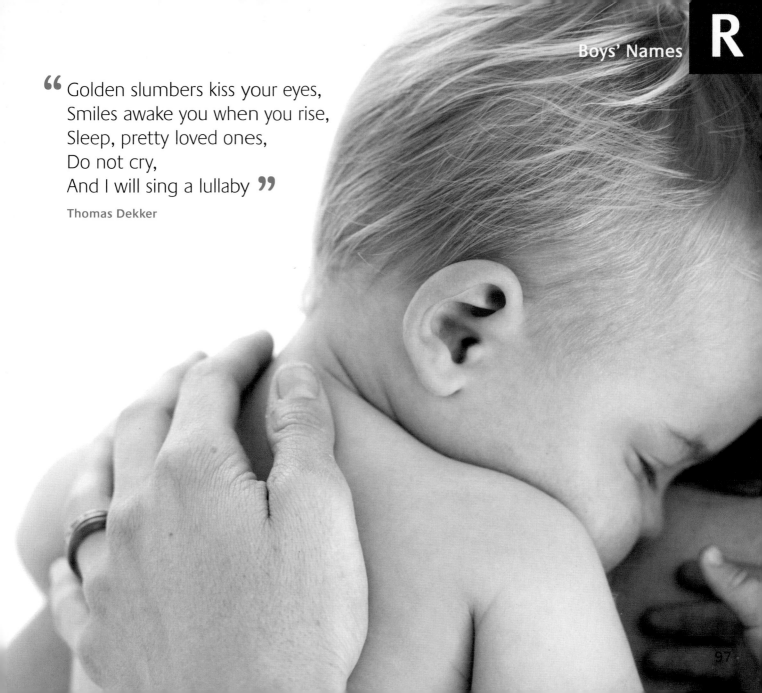

" Golden slumbers kiss your eyes,
Smiles awake you when you rise,
Sleep, pretty loved ones,
Do not cry,
And I will sing a lullaby "

Thomas Dekker

Boys' Names

Rufus
Origin/meaning: Latin 'red-haired'.
This originated as a nickname and was used by the Romans. An early example is William the Conqueror's son who was known as William Rufus, because of his red hair.
Variations and abbreviations: Rory, Roy.

Rupert
Origin/meaning: Old German 'fame-bright'.
This comes from Rupprecht, the German version of a Saxon name.
Variations: Ruppert, Rupprecht, Ruprecht.

Russell
Origin/meaning: French 'little red head'.
An aristocratic last name (it is the family name of the Duke of Bedford) it came into use as a first name in the 19th century.
Variations and abbreviations: Russ, Rusty.

Ryan
Origin/meaning: origin unclear, possibly Gaelic 'king'.
A very common Irish and English last name that is widely used now as a first name in the English-speaking world.

S

Sacha
Origin/meaning: Ancient Greek 'defender of mankind'.
A French form of Sasha, this name is now becoming popular in the English-speaking world.

Sachin
Origin/meaning: Sanskrit 'affectionate'.
A much-used name in India thanks to the huge profile of the great Indian batsman Sachin Tendulkar, one of the best cricketers in the world.

Sadiq
Origin/meaning: Arabic 'faithful'.
A popular Muslim name.
Variation: Sadiki (E African).

Said (pron. Séye-eed)

Origin/meaning: Arabic 'happy' or 'fortunate'.
A traditional Muslim name.
Variations: Saeed, Sayed.

Salim

Origin/meaning: Arabic 'peace'.
A popular Muslim name. The feminine version is Salama. 'Peace' is a traditional Muslim greeting.
Variation: Selim.

Samson

Origin/meaning: Hebrew 'child of Sham' (the sun god).
The Biblical hero Samson, with his immense strength, was the scourge of the Philistines. Delilah seduced him into revealing that his strength came from his hair, and then cut it off while he slept. The name was introduced into England at the Norman Conquest.
Variations and abbreviations: Sam, Sammy, Sampson, Sansom, Sanson (Sp), Sansone (It), Simson.

Samuel

Origin/meaning: Hebrew 'name of God'. Possibly 'Sham is God' – see Samson. Occasionally 'summer traveler', i.e. 'Viking'.
Samuel was the great prophet whose life and work is covered by the ninth and tenth books of the Old Testament. When Samuel was used in Ireland and Scotland it may have been to translate the similar Gaelic name for a Viking.
Variations and abbreviations: Sam, Sammy, Samuele (It).

Sandy

Origin/meaning: Greek 'defender of men' or 'red-haired'.
This is a familiar form of Alexander q.v. or a nickname, usually given to someone with red hair.

Sanjay

Origin/meaning: Sanskrit 'victorious'.
Sanjay Gandhi was the son of former Indian prime minister Indira Gandhi. He was killed in a plane crash in 1980.

Scott

Origin/meaning: Old English 'Scottish'.
A last name used as a first name.
Variations and abbreviations: Scot, Scotty.

Seamus (pron. Shaymus)

Origin/meaning: uncertain, possibly Hebrew 'supplanter'.
The Irish version of James or Jacob q.v.
Variations: Seumus (Scot), Shamus.

S

Boys' Names

Sean (pron. Shawn)
Origin/meaning: Hebrew 'Jehovah has favored'.
An Irish form of John q.v. through the French form Jean. It is increasingly used by non-Irish people.
Variations: Shaun, Shawn. See also John.

Sebastian
Origin/meaning: Greek 'venerable' and Latin 'from Sebastia'.
St Sebastian was particularly well known because the manner of his death (he was shot with arrows and then cudgeled to death) made a striking subject for many paintings. Shakespeare used the name for Viola's twin in his play 'Twelfth Night'.
Variations and abbreviations: Bastian, Bastien, Seb, Sebastiano (It), Sébastien (Fr), Sebastianus (Ger).

Selwyn
Origin/meaning: Old English 'friend of the house'.
An Old English name which developed as a last name. In the 19th century it came into use as a first name, perhaps influenced by the name of Bishop Selwyn who founded Selwyn College, Cambridge. It is most commonly found in Wales.
Variation: Selwin.

Sergius
Origin/meaning: uncertain. Possibly Etruscan 'fisherman'.
A popular name in Russia and other areas of the Orthodox Church because of two saints, one a Roman martyr, d.303, whose cult was very strong, and the second St Sergius of Radonegh, 1314–1392, a Russian abbot and mystic.
Variations and abbreviations: Serge, Sergé (Fr), Sergei (Russ), Sergio (It).

Seth
Origin/meaning: Hebrew 'substitute'.
This was the appropriate name given to the son born to Adam and Eve after the murder of their second son Abel, by his brother Cain.

Shane
Origin/meaning: Hebrew 'Jehovah has favored'.
An Anglicized spelling of Sean q.v. the Irish version of John.
Variation: Shan.

Shankar (pron. Sankar)
Origin/meaning: Hindu. Another name for Shiv q.v.
Shankar was a famous Hindu saint who helped defend India against Muslim invaders.

Shashi

Origin/meaning: Sanskrit 'moon'.
This can be turned into a girl's name with the addition of the suffixes -bai or -ben.

Shaun

Origin/meaning: Hebrew 'Jehovah has favored'.
An English phonetic spelling of Sean q.v.
Variation: Shawn.

Shiv (pron. Seev)

Origin/meaning: Hindu 'destruction'.
Shiv is the Lord of all creatures who supports the world by his constant meditation. Paradoxically he is also the god of death.

Shuresh (pron. Suress)

Origin/meaning: Hindu 'supreme god'.
This is an alternative name for Indra (pron. Indr). In early Hindu mythology he was the warrior king of the gods.
Variations: Surinder-Singh (Sikh), Surendra (Gujerati).

Sidney

Origin/meaning: Latin/Greek 'follower of Dionysios'.
This aristocratic last name is a contraction of St Denis, a French place name. As a first name it had the additional boost to its popularity of being the last name of the much admired Elizabethan poet Sir Philip Sidney, 1554–1586.
Variations and abbreviations: Sid, Syd, Sydney.

Siegfried

Origin/meaning: Old German 'victory peace'.
A popular German name used occasionally in Britain since the end of the 19th century. This was the direct result of the influence of Richard Wagner's opera cycle 'The Ring', in which the hero's name is Siegfried.

Silas

Origin/meaning: Latin. From Silvanus, the Roman god of uncultivated land or woodland.
Silas is close in origin to the name Silvester.
Variations and abbreviations: Si, Silvain (Fr), Silvan, Silvano (It), Silvanus (Ger/Dut), Silverio (It/Sp), Silvio (It/Sp), Sylvain (Fr), Sylvanus.

Silvester

Origin/meaning: Latin 'of the woodland'.
A name similar to Silas q.v. This was a reasonably widespread name in the Middle Ages, probably because there were three Popes who used the name.
Variations: Silvanus, Silverius, Silvestro (It), Silvius, Sylvester, Sylvestre (Fr).

Boys' Names

Simba
Origin/meaning: Swahili 'lion'.
A name familiar to the West because it was often given to lions in captivity and in literature.

Simeon
Origin/meaning: uncertain. Usually given as Hebrew 'hearkening' but may be a non-Hebrew name adopted by the Israelites. This is the usual Old Testament form of the Hebrew name Shim'on given as Simon in the New Testament.

Simon
Origin/meaning: uncertain. Usually given as Hebrew 'hearkening'. Being the Greek influenced version of the name Shim'on or Simeon it may also incorporate the Greek word meaning 'snub-nosed'. Simon owed part of its popularity to the fact that it was the original name of Peter, the head of the Apostles and the first Bishop of Rome.
Variations and abbreviations: Semjon (Russ), Si, Sim, Simeon, Siméon (Fr), Simmie, Simone (It), Simpkin, Symon, Symond (Med Eng), Ximines (Sp).

Sinclair
Origin/meaning: French. A contraction of St Clair, a town in Normandy.
This is an aristocratic last name popular as a first name in the 19th century. It is the family name of the Earls of Caithness.

Singh
Origin/meaning: Sanskrit 'lion'.
This is a Sikh name from the Punjab region. It is not used on its own but is added to other male names as a form of politeness. See also Leo and Simba.

Siôn (pron. Sheón)
Origin/meaning: Hebrew 'Jehovah has favored'.
This is the native Welsh form of John q.v.
Variation: Sionyn (dim). See also John.

Siôr (pron. Shaw)
Origin/meaning: Greek 'farmer'.
This is the Welsh form of George q.v.
Variation: Shaw.

Solomon
Origin/meaning: Hebrew 'little man of peace'.
A Biblical name referring to David's son, King Solomon, who was famous for his wisdom.
Variations and abbreviations: Salomo, Salomon (Fr/Ger), Salomón (Sp), Salomone (It), Selim (Arab), Sol, Solly, Soloman, Sulaiman (Arab). See also Salome.

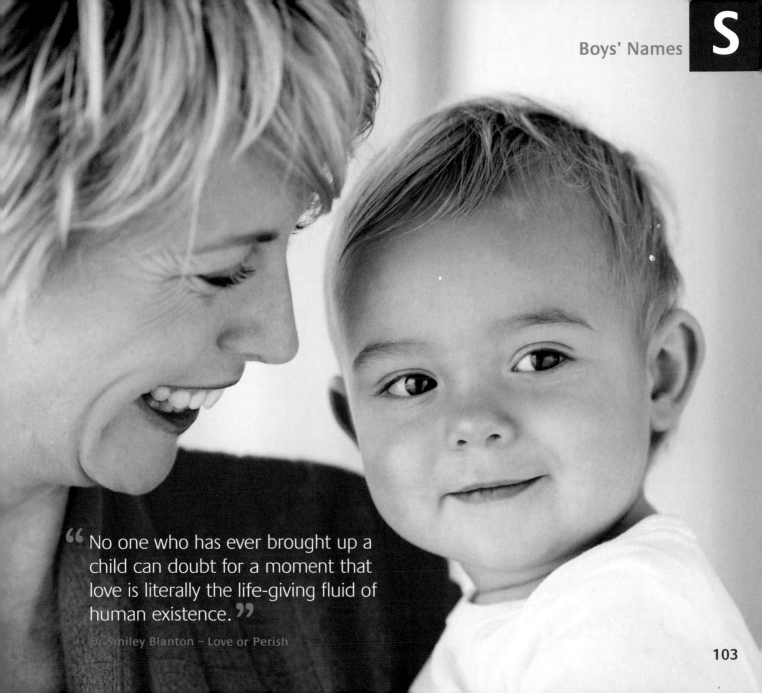

"No one who has ever brought up a child can doubt for a moment that love is literally the life-giving fluid of human existence."

Dr Smiley Blanton – Love or Perish

S

Boys' Names

Spencer

Origin/meaning: Old French 'steward' or 'butler'.

The steward was the 'dispenser' of household supplies. Used as a first name in families connected with the Spencer family and the Spencer-Churchill family (the Dukes of Marlborough), it became more widespread in the 19th century.

Variation: Spenser.

Stanley

Origin/meaning: Old English 'stony meadow'.

An aristocratic last name, the family name of the Earls of Derby, it has been used as a first name since the 19th century.

Abbreviation: Stan.

Stephen

Origin/meaning: Greek 'wreathed' or 'crowned'.

This name comes from the wreath or crown of laurel leaves given to a victorious athlete in ancient Greece. St Stephen was the first known Christian martyr who died c.35. His story is told in the Acts of the Apostles. The name was introduced into England at the Norman Conquest. Steven is an alternative spelling.

Variations and abbreviations: Etienne (Fr), Esteban (Sp), Estevan, István (Hung), Stefan (Ger/Pol), Stefano (It), Steffan (Wel), Stephan, Stéphan (Fr), Stephanus, Steve, Steven, Stevie, Stevy, Stevyn (Med Eng), Ystffan (Wel).

Stuart

Origin/meaning: Old English 'animal keeper' or 'steward'.

This Scottish last name is particularly famous as the name of the Scottish royal family. It was 1371 when one of the hereditary stewards of Scotland came to the throne as Robert II. In the 19th century Scottish last names, like aristocratic names, became generally popular.

Variations and abbreviations: Steuart, Stew, Steward, Stewart, Stu. See also Bruce, Cameron, Douglas, Graham.

Sudhakar (pron. Soothoh-kar)

Origin/meaning: Hindu 'treasure of nectar'.

The masculine equivalent of Sudha q.v.

Sulaiman

Origin/meaning: Arabic 'peaceful'.

This is a Muslim name closely related to Salim, another popular Muslim name. It is the same name as Solomon q.v.

Sven

Origin/meaning: Old Norse 'boy'.

A Scandinavian name that is now used in the English-speaking world. In Britain it is best known as the first name of the soccer manager Sven-Göran Eriksson.

T

Tad
Origin/meaning: uncertain, possibly Hebrew 'praise'.
A short form of Thaddeus q.v.

Tam
Origin/meaning: Aramaic 'twin'.
Scottish form of Thomas, as in Robert Burns' poem 'Tam O'Shanter'. It is sometimes given as an independent name.

Tancred
Origin/meaning: Old German 'grateful counsel'.
The Normans brought the name over to England in 1066, and into another of their kingdoms in Southern Italy. A famous Tancred 1078–1112 came from this kingdom of the Two Sicilies. He led the First Crusade against the Saracens in the Holy Land. In 1847 Benjamin Disraeli published a novel on the theme of Zionism called 'Tancred, The New Crusade'.
Variations: Trancrède (Fr), Trancredi (It), Tankred (Ger).

Tariq
Origin/meaning: uncertain. Possibly Arabic 'conqueror'.
Tariq was a Muslim general who led the Moorish invasion of Southern Spain.
Variation: Tarik.

Tate
Origin/meaning: Old German/Old English 'glad' or 'dear'.
An early name which developed principally as a last name, sometimes used as a first name.

Tau
Origin/meaning: Tswana 'lion'.
A name from Botswana.

Teague (pron. Theeg)
Origin/meaning: Old Irish 'poet'.
In Ireland this name developed as an easier way of saying the Old Gaelic Tadhgh. Once considered typically Irish rather as Paddy is today.
Variations and abbreviations: Teige, Thaddeus, Thaddy, Timothy.

Boys' Names

Terence
Origin/meaning: from Terentius, the name of an ancient Roman tribe. Meaning obscure. Also Old Irish 'tower of strength'. A Roman name, which like several others was used by the Irish to translate a native name, in this case, Turlough.
Variations and abbreviations: Terencio (Sp), Terenziano (It), Terenzio (It), Terrence, Terry.

Tewdwr (pron. Tudor)
Origin/meaning: The Welsh version of Theodore q.v. usually given the English spelling Tudor.

Thaddeus
Origin/meaning: uncertain, possibly Hebrew 'praise'.
In Matthew's gospel, it is given as the last name of one of the Apostles, Lebbaeus.
Variations and abbreviations: Fadej (Russ), Tad, Tadd, Taddeo (It), Tadeo (Sp), Tadeusz (Pol), Thad, Thaddoeus, Thaddäus (Ger), Thaddés (Fr), Thady.

Theobald
Origin/meaning: Old German/Old English 'bold folk'.
The medieval version of this pre-Conquest name was pronounced Tibald/t. An example of this is Tybalt, one of the characters in Shakespeare's 'Romeo and Juliet'. The common cat's name, Tibby or Tibbles, refers back to a cat named Tybalt in the medieval folk-tale cycle, 'Reynard the Fox'.
Variations and abbreviations: Dietbold (Ger), Tebaldo (It), Teobaldo (It/Sp), Thebault (Fr), Theo, Thibaud (Fr), Thibaut (Fr), Tibald, Tibold (Ger), Tiebout (Dut), Tybalt.

Theodore
Origin/meaning: Greek 'gift of God'.
Theodore Roosevelt, 1858–1919, helped to popularize the name in the US where the typical short form is Teddy. It was from Roosevelt that the Teddy bear got its name.
Variations and abbreviations: Fedor (Russ), Fyodor (Russ), Ted, Teddy, Tewdr (Wel), Teodoro (It), Theo, Théodore (Fr), Tudor (Wel). See also Jonathan, Matthew, Nathaniel.

Thomas
Origin/meaning: Aramaic 'twin'.
It was the name of one of the Apostles. The name's popularity was boosted by the reverence for St Thomas Becket. An Archbishop of Canterbury, he was killed in 1170 at the instigation of Henry II. The familiar and short forms Tommy and Tom are found in many old expressions and rhymes, e.g. 'Tom, Dick and Harry'; 'Tom, Tom, the Piper's Son'; 'Tommy' meaning private in the British army etc. All these are indications of the popularity and familiarity of the name.
Variations and abbreviations: Tam, Tamas, Tammie, Tammy, Thom, Tom, Tómás (Sp), Tomas (Ir), Tomaso (It), Tompkin, Tommie, Tommy.

Thurstan

Origin/meaning: Old Norse/Old English 'Thor's stone'.

A last name from East Anglia which is also used as a first name. Sometimes said to be the origin of the name Tristram q.v.

Variations: Thurston, Tristram.

Timothy

Origin/meaning: Greek 'honor to God'.

This is a Greek name pre-dating Christianity. It was the name of St Paul's companion in the Acts of the Apostles. Although it is now a very familiar name it did not come into use until the period of Biblical names after the Protestant Reformation, when it became popular with English and American Puritans.

Variations and abbreviations: Tim, Timmie, Timmy, Timoteo (It/Sp), Timothée (Fr), Timotheus (Ger/Dut).

Titus

Origin/meaning: uncertain, possibly Greek 'honored'.

A Latin name, derived from the Greek. One of the followers of St Paul, to whom he wrote one of his Epistles, was called Titus.

Variation: Tito (It).

Tobias

Origin/meaning: Hebrew 'God is good'.

The more familiar English form is Toby q.v. Tobias was the son of Tobit in the Book of Tobit (Apocrypha).

Toby

Origin/meaning: Hebrew 'God is good'.

The English form of Tobiah, generally more popular than the Greek form, Tobias q.v. The Book of Tobit (omitted from the Authorized Version of the Bible) was a popular Biblical story in the Middle Ages and tells the story of the pious Tobit and his son Tobias. Other indications of the popularity of the name are its use for Mr Punch's dog (in the Bible Tobias owned a dog) and for the Toby jug.

Variations and abbreviations: Tobia (It), Tobiah, Tobias (Ger), Tobie (Fr), Tobin, Tobit.

Tom

Origin/meaning: Aramaic 'twin'.

A common short form of Thomas, often used as an independent name.

Tony

Origin/meaning: Latin Antonius – the name of one of the great Roman families.

The most popular short form of Antony q.v. sometimes given as an independent name.

T

Boys' Names

Torquil
Origin/meaning: obscure, possibly Old Norse 'Thor's cauldron'.
This is the Gaelic version of an Old Norse name introduced into Scotland and the North of England by the Vikings from the 8th–11th centuries.
Variations: Thorkill, Thorketill, Torcull.

Travis
Origin/meaning: Old French 'toll collector'.
An occupation name now used as a first name. Its popularity has been boosted by the success of pop group Travis.

Trevor
Origin/meaning: Old Welsh 'large settlement'.
This is a Welsh place name which is found as a given name or last name as far back as the 10th century. The Welsh form is Trefor.
Abbreviation: Trev.

Trey
Origin/meaning: Old English 'three' or 'third born'.
Mostly found in the US.

Tristan
Origin/meaning: uncertain. Either Old Welsh 'herald', Latin/French 'sad' or Old Norse 'Thor's stone'.
Variation: Tristano (It).

Tristram
Origin/meaning: uncertain. Either Old Welsh 'herald', Latin 'sad' or Old Norse 'Thor's stone'.
There may be an element of all these definitions in Tristram for the name seems to have developed independently in several countries. Tristram and Iseult (Tristan and Isolde) is an Arthurian romance which may date back as far as the 6th century.
Variations: Thurstan, Tristan (Fr), Tristano (It), Tristran, Trystram.

Troy
Origin/meaning: Old Irish 'foot soldier' or a place name after Troy in Asia Minor or Troyes in France.
Town names from the ancient Greek world were often given to settlements in North America after the civil war as if to emphasize the influence of Greek democracy. For the same reason these city names were sometimes used as personal names.

Truman
Origin/meaning: Old German, Old English 'true man'.
A name largely found in the US and whose use was boosted by the example of US president Harry S. Truman, 1884–1972.
Variation: Trueman.

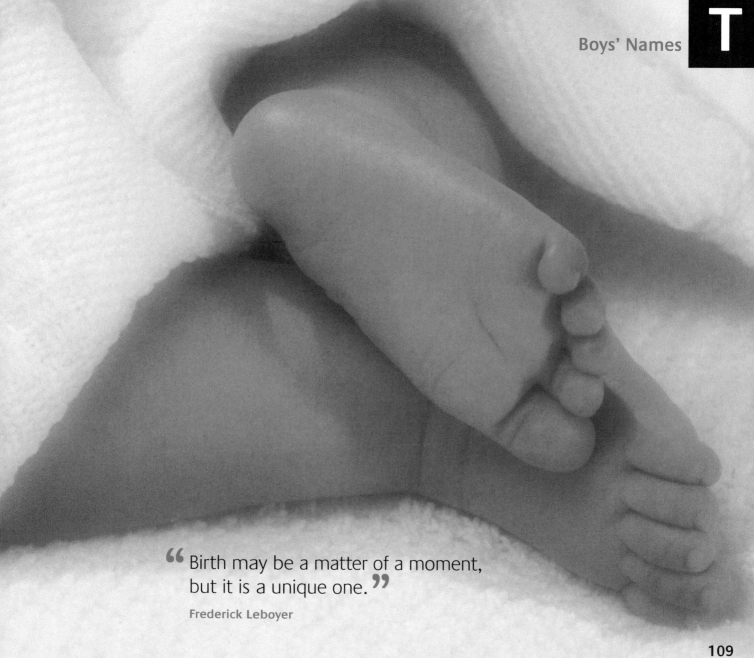

"Birth may be a matter of a moment, but it is a unique one."

Frederick Leboyer

Boys' Names

Ty
Origin/meaning: a short form of names beginning with Ty. Most are last names used as first names, e.g. Tyler, Tynan.

Tyler
Origin/meaning: English 'roof tiler'.
This occupational name is very popular now, especially in the US. It is also used as a name for girls.
Variations: Ty, Tyla.

Tyrone
Origin/meaning: Old Irish 'land of Owen'.
This is an Irish place name (County Tyrone), and an aristocratic last name – the Earl of Tyrone is the elder son of the Marquess of Waterford.

U

Ulysses
Origin/meaning: uncertain, possibly Etruscan 'wanderer'. Sometimes given as 'hater'. In Ireland 'mind reward'.
This is the Latin form of Odysseus, the name of a Geek hero of the Trojan wars whose journeyings are described in Homer's epic poem 'The Odyssey'. In Ireland it was used to translate the native names Ulrick and Uileos. The Irish writer James Joyce used it as the title of one of his novels published in 1922. In the US it has been used to honor Ulysses S. Grant.
Variations and abbreviations: Uileos, Uillioc (Ir), Ulick (Ir), Ulises (Sp), Ulisse (It).

Umar
Origin/meaning: Arabic 'highest'. Sanskrit 'husband of Uma'.
This is another name for Shiv q.v. (Lord Shiva) as Uma was a reincarnation of Parvati q.v., Shiva's wife.

Uni
Origin/meaning: Yao 'life'.
A name from Malawi in Central Africa.

Uriah
Origin/meaning: Hebrew 'light of Jehovah'.
This is a Biblical name used occasionally by Puritans after the 16th-century Protestant Reformation.

V

Valentine

Origin/meaning: Latin 'strong', 'healthy'.
Well known because of St Valentine the Roman martyr, whose feast day (February 14th) coincided with a pagan festival in which young people chose partners. This tradition was retained by the new Christian religion.
Variations and abbreviations: Val, Valentijn (Dut), Valentin (Fr/Ger/Scand/Sp), Valentine (It).

Vere

Origin/meaning: 'from Ver' (an area of Normandy).
A last name introduced at the Conquest. Its aristocratic connections made it an ideal candidate for adoption as a first name during the 19th century.

Vernon

Origin/meaning: Latin 'springlike' or Old French 'little alder grove'.
Either a masculine form of the Latin word Verna or a typical 19th-century adoption of an aristocratic last name.
Variations and abbreviations: Vern, Verne, Verney.

Vidal

Origin/meaning: Latin 'vital' or 'belonging to life'.
A Spanish form of the rare English name Vitalis. A more current English equivalent of Vivian q.v.

Vijay

Origin/meaning: Sanskrit 'victory'.
Variation: Viajay.

Vikram/a (the final a is not pronounced)

Origin/meaning: Sanskrit 'a record-breaker'.
Vikram, whose full title was Vikramaditya (Vikram of the eternal) was a legendary Indian Raja (king) possibly based on the real King Chandragupta II, 375–415. From the gods Vikram received the power of flight and the ability to communicate with animals and birds.

Vinay

Origin/meaning: Hindu 'courtesy'.

Boys' Names

Vincent

Origin/meaning: Latin 'conquering'.
This name was used in Medieval England to honor St Vincentius of Saragossa who was martyred by the Emperor Diocletian at the beginning of the 4th century. In later centuries the reputation of St Vincent de Paul, 1576–1660, made Vincent a popular name with Catholics in many European countries.
Variations and abbreviations: Vicente (Sp), Vin, Vince, Vincente, Vincenzo (It), Vinny, Vinzent, Vinzenz (Ger).

Vishnu

Origin/meaning: Hindu. The name of one of the greatest of the Hindu gods.
According to the Hindu religion Vishnu is probably the greatest of all the gods, although he himself acknowledged the supremacy of Shiva. At crucial points in the cycle of time Vishnu is incarnated and comes to earth.

Vivian

Origin/meaning: Latin 'full of life'.
A rare masculine name which, as Vivianus, dates back to the early Middle Ages.
Variations and abbreviations: Viv, Vivien (Fr), Viviano (It), Vyvyan.

Vladimir

Origin/meaning: Slavic 'famous prince'.
Prince and saint, Vladimir, 955–1015, is credited with the definite conversion of European Russia to Christianity.

W

Walid

Origin/meaning: Arabic 'new born'.
This is a Muslim name.
Variation: Waleed.

Wallace

Origin/meaning: Old Scots 'from Wales' or 'Welsh'.
A famous Scottish last name initially used as a first name in the 19th century when aristocratic last names were fashionable.
Variations and abbreviations: Wal, Wally.

Walter

Origin/meaning: Old German/Old English 'rule-people'.

The Norman version of this name was very popular. One of the most popular short forms Wat, indicates that in the Middle Ages the pronunciation was Water.
Variations and abbreviations: Gauthier (Fr), Gautier, Gaulterio (Sp), Gualtiero (It), Gwaleter (Wel), Wally, Walt, Walther (Ger), Wat.

Waqar
Origin/meaning: Arabic 'dignity'.
A popular name in Pakistan.
Variation: Waqaar.

Warren
Origin/meaning: probably Old German 'of the Verini tribe'. Sometimes listed as 'defender'.
Warren developed almost exclusively into a last name in the Middle Ages. Its use as a first name has been revived in the last 100 years, particularly in America.

Wasim
Origin/meaning: Arabic 'handsome'.
Wasim Akram was an extremely talented Pakistani cricketer in the 1980s and 1990s.
Variation: Waseem.

Washington
Origin/meaning: Old English 'home of the Wassa folk'.
Washington in County Durham gave its name to the family of George Washington, first President of the US. As a result this last name has periodically been popular as a first name in the US.

Wayne
Origin/meaning: Old English 'wagon'.
A last name, sometimes a short form of Wainwright (wagon-mender). Frequently found as a first name in the US because of film actor John Wayne and the hero of the Revolution General Anthony Wayne.

Wilbur
Origin/meaning: either Old German 'resolute defence' or Dutch 'wild farmer'.
This name, so popular in the US but rare in other English-speaking countries, may have either or both of the above meanings. In both cases it derives from a last name.
Variations and abbreviations: Will, Wilber.

Wilfred
Origin/meaning: Old English 'will peace', i.e. 'determined for peace'.
This Old English name usually found before 1066 as Wilfrith, did not survive the competition of the new names which arrived with the Conquest. It was revived in the 19th century.
Variations and abbreviations: Fred, Wilf, Wilfrid, Will.

William

Origin/meaning: Old German 'will helmet', i.e. 'helmet of resolution'.
One of the most consistently popular names in England since it was introduced in the old forms Wilhelm and Guillamo by William the Conqueror in 1066. Will used to be the most common short form but in the last few hundred years Bill and Billy have become more popular.
Variations and abbreviations: Bill, Billie, Billy, Guglielmo (It), Guillaume (Fr), Guillermo (Sp), Gwylim (Wel), Liam (Ir), Vilhelm (Scand/Slav), Wilhelm (Ger), Will, Willem (Dut), Willie, Willis.

Winston

Origin/meaning: Old English 'friend's farm' (the name of a small village in Gloucestershire).
The family name of the grandmother of John Churchill, 1st Duke of Marlborough, and it is still a regularly used name in the Churchill family. Sir Winston Churchill was a grandson of the 7th Duke of Marlborough.
Variations and abbreviations: Win, Winnie, Winny.

Wolfgang

Origin/meaning: Old German 'approach of the wolf'.
A South German/Austrian name world famous because of the Austrian composer Wolfgang Amadeus Mozart, 1756–1791.
Variations and abbreviations: Volfango (It), Wolf, Wolfe, Wolfie, Wolfy, Wulf.

Wyatt

Origin/meaning: Old English 'battle strong'.
The best-known bearer of this name was the famous US lawman Wyatt Earp.

Wynne

Origin/meaning: Welsh 'white/fair'.
A form of Gwyn q.v. It is found as part of many Welsh names as well as being a name in its own right.

X

Xavier (pron. Sp Havierr, Eng Zayvier).

Origin/meaning: Arabic 'bright' or 'splendid'.
The last name of the Spanish missionary St Francis Xavier, 1506–1552. It is a popular name among Catholics, particularly of course in Spanish-speaking countries.
Variations: Javier, Xaver (Ger).

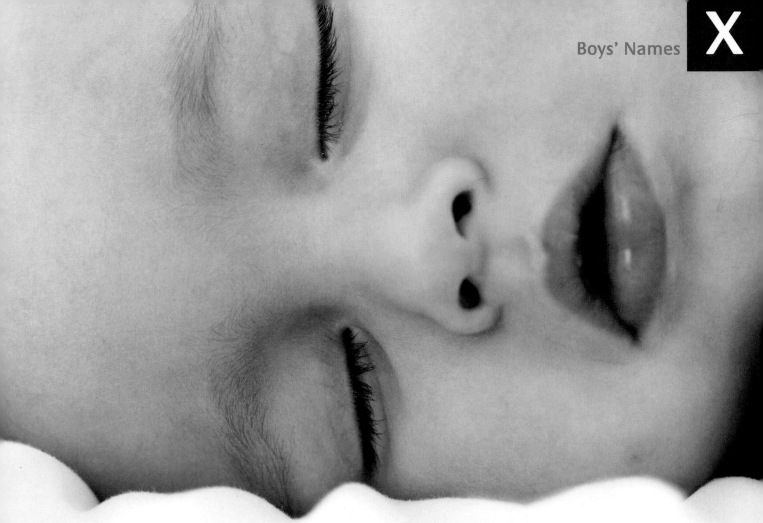

66 The smile that flickers on baby's lips when he sleeps – does anybody know where it was born? Yes, there is a rumour that a young pale beam of a crescent moon touched the edge of a vanishing autumn cloud, and there the first smile was first born in the dream of a dew-washed morning. 99

Rabindranath Tagore, Gitanjali, no 61.

Boys' Names

Ximenes (pron. Sp Hímehnehth, Eng Ziminez)
Origin/meaning: Hebrew 'hearkening'.
A Spanish form of Simon q.v.

Yaqub
Origin/meaning: Arabic 'supplanter'.
This is the same name as the Hebrew Jacob and English James.

Yehudi
Origin/meaning: Hebrew 'praise of the Lord'.
A Jewish form of Jude q.v. as is Judah.
Variations and abbreviations: see Jude.

Yestin
Origin/meaning: Latin 'just'.
The Welsh version of Justin.
Variation: Iestin.

Yogesh (pron. Yogess)
Origin/meaning: Sanskrit/Gujerati 'expert at yoga'.

Yusuf
Origin/meaning: Arabic 'he shall add (to his power)'.
This is the Muslim form of the Hebrew name Joseph q.v.

Yves (pron. Eve)
Origin/meaning: Old German 'yew'.
The French version of the English Ivo or Ives, common in Medieval France, particularly in Brittany, and still popular today.
Variation: Yvon.

Z

Zacchaeus

Origin/meaning: Hebrew 'the Lord has remembered'.

The Latinized version of the short form of Zachariah (see Zachary). Zacchaeus (Luke 19) was a small man, a publican, who climbed a sycamore tree to get a good view of Jesus.

Zachary

Origin/meaning: Hebrew 'the Lord has remembered'.

This is the English version of the Biblical name Zachariah or Zacharias. It is still found in the US, particularly in one of its short forms.

Variations and abbreviations: Zacarias (Sp), Zaccaria (It), Zacharias, Zachariah, Zacharian, Zacharie (Fr), Zack, Zacky, Zak, Zechariah, Zeke.

Zaid

Origin/meaning: Arabic 'increase'.

A common Muslim name.

Variations: Zaeed, Zayed, Ziyad.

Zavier (pron. Záyvyer)

Origin/meaning: Arabic 'bright'.

One of the Anglicized versions of Xavier q.v.

Variation: Zaver.

Zebedee

Origin/meaning: Hebrew 'gift of the Lord'.

Zebedee was the father of the Apostles James and John (Mark ch.1:19).

Variations and abbreviations: Zeb, Zebadiah, Zebediah.

Zeke

Origin/meaning: Hebrew 'the Lord has remembered' or Hebrew 'God is strong'.

A short form of Zachary or Ezekial, found as an independent name in the US.

A

Aakash (pron. Akass)
Origin/meaning: Hindu 'sky'.
Found throughout India but considered rather unusual.

Aarti
Origin/meaning: Hindu.
The name of a prayer made with a candle. This name comes from West India.

Abbey, Abby
Origin/meaning: Hebrew 'father of joy'.
Popular North American contraction of Abigail q.v. used as a name in its own right.

Abebi
Origin/meaning: Yoruba 'asked for child'.
A Nigerian name. Abeje and Abeke have similar meanings.

Abigail
Origin/meaning: Hebrew 'father's joy' or 'father (source) of joy'.
One of the wives of King David. In the 17th-century play 'The Scornful Lady' by Beaumont and Fletcher, Abigail was the handmaid and confidante of the heroine. As a result Abigail became synonymous with maid servant.
Variations and abbreviations: Abigael, Abagail, Abaigael (Ir), Abbe, Abbi, Abbie, Abby, Abbye, Abigael, Gael, Gail, Gale, Gayel, Gayle.

Acacia
Origin/meaning: Greek 'guileless, innocent', 'acacia tree'.
The acacia tree is said to symbolize the resurrection and therefore immortality.
Variations and abbreviations: Cacia, Cacie, Casey.

Ada
Origin/meaning: Old German Eda, Etta and Old English Eadda, 'happy'.
Popular in Britain in the 18th and 19th centuries. Byron's first daughter, the mathematician, b.1816, was christened Ada.

Adela
Origin/meaning: 'noble' from the Old German 'adal'.

Adela was brought over to England at the time of the Norman Conquest. It enjoyed a period of popularity in the 19th century partly because of the fashionable French version Adèle.
Variations and abbreviations: Ad, Adel, Adèle (Fr), Adella, Adelle, Addie. See also Adelaide, Adeline, Alice.

Adelaide

Origin/meaning: Old German 'nobility'.
The original Old German version was Adalheid. Old French corrupted Adalheid to Adeliz from which we get Alice q.v. Adelaide, the French version, became popular in England soon after the accession to the throne in 1830 of William IV and his wife Queen Adelaide. The capital of the state of South Australia was named Adelaide after the Queen in 1836.
Variations and abbreviations: Ada, Adalheid, Addi, Addie, Adel, Adelaida (Ital), Adelheid (Ger), Della, Heidi (Ger). See also Adela, Adeline, Alice.

Adeline

Origin/meaning: Old German 'nobility', 'noble maiden'.
This has the same root, 'adal' – 'noble', as Adela and Adelaide. They were all brought to Britain with the Norman Conquest.
Variations and abbreviations: Addi, Addy, Adel, Adelena, Adelene, Adelina (Ital), Aline q.v., Edelina, Edolina.

Adeola

Origin/meaning: Yoruba 'crown has honor'.
A Nigerian name. One of several similar names such as Adedagbo – 'happiness is a crown', and Adeleke – 'crown achieves happiness'.

Aditi

Origin/meaning: Hindu. Meaning obscure.
In mythology Aditi was one of the wives of the Hindu saint Kasnyapa. She gave birth to all the gods.

Adriana/Adrienne

Origin/meaning: Latin 'from Adria'.
Feminine versions of Adrian, q.v.
Variations and abbreviations: Adria, Adriane (Ger), Adrianna, Adrianne, Hadria.

Aduke (pron. Adóokay)

Origin/meaning: Yoruba 'much loved child'.
A name from Nigeria.

Afiya

Origin/meaning: Swahili 'health'.
An East African name.

A

Girls' Names

Afra
Origin/meaning: obscure. May be Latin 'African', an abbreviation of Greek, Aphrodite, or Hebrew 'house of dust'. There is a 4th-century saint called Afra, whose feast day is August 5th.
Variations: Aphra, Ayfara, Aphry.

Agatha
Origin/meaning: Ancient Greek 'good'.
The name of a 3rd-century Sicilian Saint, Agatha was a popular medieval name. William the Conqueror gave it to one of his daughters.

Agnes
Origin/meaning: Greek 'pure', chaste.
This was an extremely popular name during the Middle Ages and was found in a variety of forms. One of these, Annis, shows us how it used to be pronounced.
Variations and abbreviations: Aggi, Aggie, Agna, Agnella, Agnese (Ital), Agneta (Scand), Agnete (Ital), Annis (Med Eng), Annys, Ines (Sp), Inez, Nezza, Nessie, Nesta (Wel), Ynes, Ynez. See also Senga.

Aida (pron. Ayéeda)
Origin/meaning: Arabic 'benefit'.
This name is quite separate from Aida, a version of Ada q.v.

Aileen
Origin/meaning: Greek 'light' or 'bright'.
The Irish version of the immensely popular name Helen.
Variations: Ailene, Aleen, Ailene, Eileen, Ilene, Ileana.

Ailsa
Origin/meaning: uncertain. Possibly Hebrew 'God is my satisfaction' or Old German 'noble'.
This is almost exclusively Scottish and may simply be a native Scottish name with no certain meaning.

Aithne (pron. Ethnee or Awnye)
Origin/meaning: Old Irish 'little fire', 'little fiery one'.
The feminine version of Aidan q.v. In Irish mythology Aine (pron. Awnye) was Queen of the Fairies.
Variations and abbreviations: Aine (Old Celtic), Eithne, Ena, Ethne, Ina.

Aiyetoro (pron. Aryétoro)
Origin/meaning: Yoruba 'peace on earth'.
This name comes from East Africa.

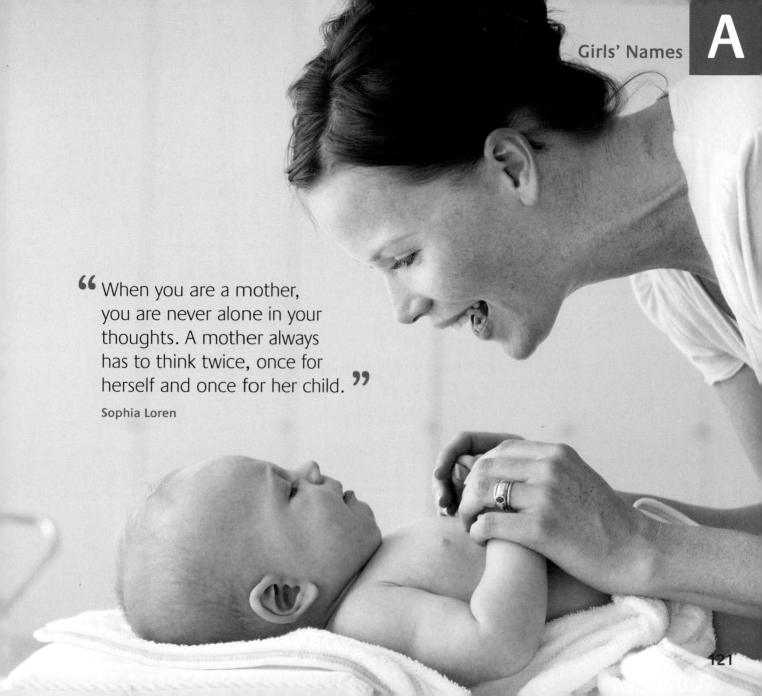

"When you are a mother, you are never alone in your thoughts. A mother always has to think twice, once for herself and once for her child."

Sophia Loren

A

Girls' Names

Alanna
Origin/meaning: Celtic 'beautiful'.
The feminine form of Alan q.v.
Variations and abbreviations: Alaine, Alana, Alanda, Alane, Alayne, Alina, Allene, Allin, Allina, Allyn, Lana, Lanna.

Alba
Origin/meaning: Latin 'white', 'blonde'.
Variation: Alva.

Alberta
Origin/meaning: Old German 'nobly bright'.
Feminine version of Albert q.v.
Variations and abbreviations: Adalberta (Old Ger), Albertina (Ital), Albertine (Fr), Ally, Elberta, Elbertina, Elbertine, Berta, Bartie.

Alcina
Origin/meaning: Greek 'sea-maiden'.
Variations: Alcine, Alcinia.

Alethea
Origin/meaning: Greek 'truth'.
Like other virtues, Faith, Hope, Prudence etc., Alethea was a popular name in the Puritan England of the 17th century and among Puritan settlers in America.
Variations and abbreviations: Alatheia, Aleta, Aletea (Sp), Alethia, Aletia, Aletta, Alithia.

Alexandra
Origin/meaning: Greek 'defender of men'.
The feminine form of Alexander q.v. The name achieved popularity in English-speaking countries in the 19th century with the marriage of the Prince of Wales, later Edward VII, to Princess Alexandra of Denmark in 1863.
Variations and abbreviations: Alejandra (Sp), Alessandra (Ital), Alex, Alexa, Alexandria, Alexandrina, Alexina, Alexine, Alexis, Ali, Alix, Alla, Alli, Lexi, Lexine, Sandi, Sandie, Sandra, Sandy, Sondra, Zandra, Zandria.

Alguni
Origin/meaning: Hindu: the name of the 5th month of the year.
In this month there is a big religious festival in West and North India, which celebrates the arrival of Spring.

Alice
Origin/meaning: Old German 'nobility' or Greek 'truth'.
It comes from the Norman French version of Adelaide – Adelize. When this name was translated into Latin in documents it

became Alesia from which Alice eventually developed. Very popular in the Middle Ages, usually as Alys. Its popularity was greatly increased by the success of Lewis Carroll's book 'Alice's Adventures in Wonderland', published in 1865.
Variations and abbreviations: Adelice, Adelize, Ali, Alicea, Alis, Alisa, Alison, Allison, Allyce, Allys, Alyss, Alyssa.

Aline
Origin/meaning: Old German 'nobility' from adal 'noble'.
Short form of Adeline q.v. Often used as an independent name. Sometimes confused with Aileen, the Irish form of Helen.
Variations: Alena, Alene, Alina, Alyna, Arleen, Arline.

Alison
Origin/meaning: Old German 'nobility'.
A diminutive form of Alice q.v. which is itself a derivation of Adelaide q.v. It is now an independent first name.
Variations and abbreviations: Alicen, Allison, Alyson, Elsie.

Allegra
Origin/meaning: Italian 'cheerful'.
An Italian name. Given to Lord Byron's daughter by his mistress Claire Clairmont.

Alma
Origin/meaning: Latin 'kind' or Italian 'soul'.
This name enjoyed a vogue after the Battle of Alma, 1854, which was an incident in the Crimean War.

Almeria
Origin/meaning: Arabic 'princess'.

Almira
Origin/meaning: Arabic 'truth'.
Variation: Elmira.

Alphonsine
Origin/meaning: Old German 'noble and ready'.
A French feminine form of Alphonse, comparatively recent in origin.
Variations: Alfonsina (Ital), Alfonsine, Alonsa, Alonza.

Althea
Origin/meaning: Greek 'wholesome'.

A

Girls' Names

Aluna (pron. Alóona)
Origin/meaning: 'come here'.
A name used in Kenya.

Alyssa
Origin/meaning: Greek 'sane', 'wise'; also the name of a yellow rock plant, alyssum.
This may be an independent name or it can be regarded as a form of Alice q.v.

Amanda
Origin/meaning: Latin 'lovable'.
Another of the many names which originate from the Latin verb 'amare' – 'to love'.
Amanda seems to have begun as a contrived name in the 17th century when names were made up to underline the personalities of characters in the plays of the time.
Variations and abbreviations: Manda, Mandie, Mandy.

Amarylis (pron. Ammahrýllis)
Origin/meaning: Ancient Greek 'fresh stream'.
Used by the Greek and Roman poets as a name for a fresh country girl. In the 17th century English poets such as Milton, taking up the current fashion for giving characters names which expressed their virtues, used it in their own poetry.

Amber
Origin/meaning: Arabic/French. The name given to a translucent yellow resin used as a semi-precious stone.
This name was only rarely used before the book 'Forever Amber' by Kathleen Winsor, which was a best-seller in the 1950s.

Amelia
Origin/meaning: Old German 'hard work', 'industrious'.
The original Old German name Amalburga became Amelie in France. Amelia is the Latinized version which the Hanoverians brought to England in the 18th century.
Variations and abbreviations: Amalea, Amalia (Ital), Ameliarane, Amalie (Ger), Amelie (Fr), Amilia (Scot), Amiline, Emilia, Emelina, Emiline, Emily, Emmeline.

Amina
Origin/meaning: Arabic 'honest', 'faithful'.
A very popular Muslim and North African name.
Variation: Aminah. See Sati.

Amrita
Origin/meaning: Sanskrit 'immortal'.

In the Hindu texts, the ocean is churned to create ambrosia – from which the name Amrita derives – which when drunk allows the gods to defeat the demons.

Amy

Origin/meaning: Latin/French 'beloved'.

Amy became popular because of the 13th-century St Amata. Like many medieval names it enjoyed a 19th-century revival especially after Sir Walter Scott's book 'Kenilworth' about the Earl of Leicester's ill-fated wife Amy Robsart.

Variations: Aimée (Fr), Aimie, Amata (Ir/Sp), Ame, Ami, Amia, Amya, Amye, Anwyl (Wel), Esmé.

Anastasia

Origin/meaning: Greek 'resurrection'.

The name of a 4th-century saint who was martyred in Yugoslavia. Anastasia has always been more popular in Greece and Russia than in the West. The Grand Duchess Anastasia, daughter of Czar Nicholas II of Russia, is claimed to have escaped from the Bolsheviks who executed the rest of her family in 1918.

Variations and abbreviations: Amstice, Ana, Anastasie (Fr), Anstice, Nastasia (It), Nastasya (Russ), Stace, Stacey, Stacie, Stacy.

Andrea

Origin/meaning: Greek 'manly', 'brave'.

A Latinized feminine form of Andrew (which was originally used for girls as well as boys).

Angela

Origin/meaning: Greek 'messenger'.

Angel was the word used to translate the Hebrew word for messenger of God and it was occasionally used as a masculine name. The feminine form was first found as a proper name in the 16th and 17th centuries.

Variations: Angèle (Fr), Angelia, Angelica.

Angharad

Origin/meaning: Old Welsh 'much loved'.

Anila

Origin/meaning: Sanskrit 'air, wind'.

The feminine form of Anil. In the Hindu text, Vedas, Anil is the name of the wind god (also known as Vayu) who drove a golden chariot pulled by a thousand horses.

Anita

Origin/meaning: Hebrew 'graceful', 'little graceful one'.

A Spanish and Italian diminutive form of Ann q.v.

Variation and abbreviation: Nita.

Girls' Names

Anju
Origin/meaning: Sanskrit 'one who lives in heart'.

Ann, Anne
Origin/meaning: Hebrew 'graceful'.
Ann and its variations are all based on the Hebrew name Hannah q.v. St Anne was popularly supposed to be the mother of the Virgin Mary. The name came to the West from the Byzantine Empire via Russia at about the time of the Norman Conquest. By the 17th century it was one of the most common English names. The accession of Queen Anne to the English throne in 1701 confirmed its popularity.
Variations and abbreviations: Ana, Anette, Anja (Russ), Anita (Sp/It), Anna (Ger/It/Dut/Scand), Annetta, Annette (Fr), Anni, Annie, Anny, Anouska (Russ), Anya (Russ), Nan, Nana, Nancy, Nannie, Nita.

Anna
Origin/meaning: Hebrew 'graceful'.
A Latin form of Ann which became popular in England in the 18th century.

Annabel
Origin/meaning: Latin/French 'lovable'.
This name is Scottish and dates from the 12th century. There is no convincing evidence for the frequent assumption that it is a combination of Anna and Bella, meaning 'beautiful Ann', as it appears in Scotland well before the name Anne.
Variations and abbreviations: Annabella (It), Annabelle, Annabla (Ir), Bella, Belle. See also Arabella.

Annunciata
Origin/meaning: Latin 'bearer of news'.
This is a name which refers to the occasion when the Virgin Mary was told by an angel that she was to be the Mother of Jesus, celebrated in the Catholic Church on March 25th. The name is therefore given to girls born in March.
Variations: Annunziata (It), Annunciacion (Sp), Maria Annunciata (It).

Anthea
Origin/meaning: Greek 'flowery'.
One of the 17th-century literary names created to give characters names appropriate to their appearance or personality. See also Flora, Fleur.

Antonia
Origin/meaning: from the Latin name Antonius, one of the Patrician families of Ancient Rome. Sometimes considered to mean 'inestimable' or 'priceless'. A feminine form of Antony q.v.
Variations and abbreviations: Anthoine (Fr), Antoinette (Fr), Antonetta (Scand), Antonie (Ger), Antonietta (It), Antonina (It), Netta, Nettie, Netty, Toni, Tonia, Tonie, Tony.

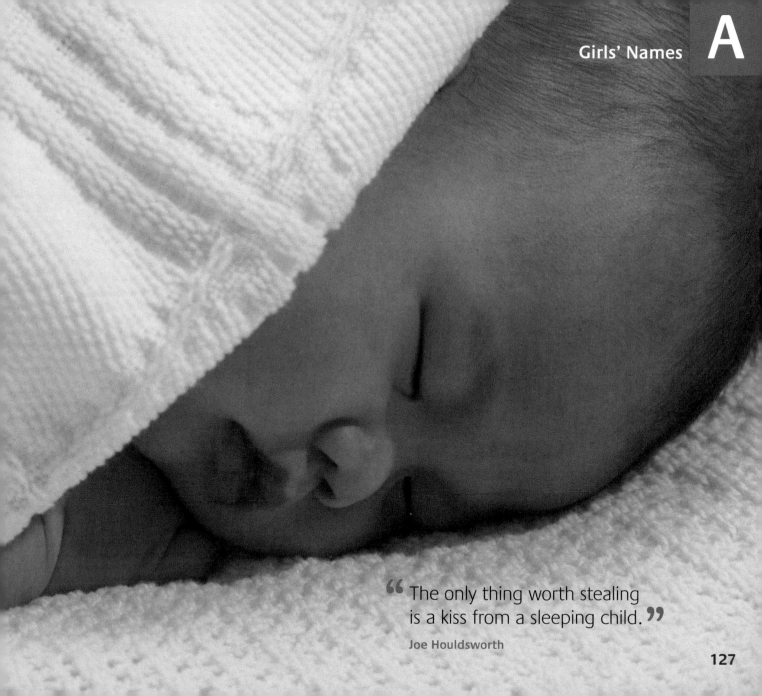

❝The only thing worth stealing
is a kiss from a sleeping child.❞

Joe Houldsworth

Girls' Names

Apple
Origin/meaning: English, the name of the fruit.
First known as a given name when used by Hollywood actress Gwyneth Paltrow for her daughter.

April
Origin/meaning: Latin 'opening', 'beginning of Spring'. The name of the fourth month of the year.
A comparatively recent 20th-century name.
Variation: Avril (Fr).

Arabella
Origin/meaning: Latin 'lovable'.
This name was originally found only in Scotland and dates from the 12th century.

Araminta
Origin/meaning: Latin 'loving'.
This name was one of many made-up names found in 17th-century literature, which were taken up and used by real people.
Variation: Aminta.

Ardelle
Origin/meaning: Latin 'warm, enthusiastic'.
Variations and abbreviations: Arad, Ardelia, Ardella, Ardene, Ardine.

Ariadne
Origin/meaning: Greek 'very holy one'.
Originally the name of the daughter of the mythological King Minos of Crete. She helped Theseus escape from the labyrinth where the Minotaur was waiting to kill him, by giving him a ball of silk to mark his route.
Variations: Ariane (Fr/Ger), Ariana, Arianna (It).

Arianwen
Origin/meaning: Old Welsh 'silver white'.
See also Alba, Blanche.

Armine
Origin/meaning: Old German 'army person', 'a soldier'.
Rare feminine version of Armin, an English form of Armand. The variation Arminel is found in the Devon area of England.
Variations: Armina, Arminda, Arminel, Arminie, Armande (Fr).

Aruna
Origin/meaning: Sanskrit 'reddish-brown'.
The feminine form of Arun who, in Hindu texts, is the personification of dawn. Aruna is also the name of a number of plants including bitter apple.

Arwa
Origin/meaning: Arabic 'mountain goats'.
A name popular in the Gulf States as well as Saudi Arabia and Jordan.

Asha
Origin/meaning: Sanskrit 'hope'.
In Hindu texts, Asha is the wife of one of the eight Vasus (demi-gods).

Asmita (pron. Asméeta)
Origin/meaning: Hindu 'self-respect'.
Found throughout India.

Astrid
Origin/meaning: Old Norse 'God's strength'.
Used by Scandinavian Royal families since the 11th century when it was the name of the wife of the Norwegian King and saint, Olaf.
Variations and abbreviations: Asta, Assa, Assi, Atti, Estrid.

Atalanta
Origin/meaning: Greek 'swift runner'.
In Greek mythology Atalanta was an athlete who would only marry someone who ran faster than she could. Suitors who lost the race were killed. Hippomenes was given three golden apples by the goddess Aphrodite which he placed in Atalanta's path. He then won the race because she stopped en route to pick up the golden apples.
Variations: Atalante, Allante, Atlanta, Tala.

Athena
Origin/meaning: Greek 'wisdom'.
Athena was the Greek goddess of wisdom. Her symbol was an owl. Athens was named in her honor and was under her protection.
Variation: Athene (Fr).

Audrey
Origin/meaning: Old English 'noble strength'.
Audrey is a contraction of Ethelreda. After 1000 years Audrey became common as an independent name in the 16th century. The word tawdry comes from the name because of the lace and other cheap ornaments sold at St Ethelreda's fair on the Isle of Ely where the 7th-century saint of that name had founded an abbey.
Variations and abbreviations: Audi, Audie, Audrie, Audry, Audrye, Dee. See also Adelaide, Alice.

A

Girls' Names

Augusta

Origin/meaning: Latin 'venerable', 'majestic'. Title given to female relations of the Roman emperors.
Feminine version of Augustus q.v. The Hanoverians brought both the masculine and feminine versions to England in the 18th century and Augusta became popular in the 19th century. Sometimes used for girls born in the month of August which is itself named after the Roman Emperor, Augustus.
Variations and abbreviations: Auguste (Dut/Fr/Ger/Scand), Augustina, Augustine, Austina, Austine, Gus, Gussie, Gussy, Tina.

Aurora

Origin/meaning: Latin 'dawn'.
In Roman mythology Aurora was the goddess of the dawn. It is one of many classical names revived during the Renaissance and popularized by 17th-century literature. Oriana q.v. may be a version of the same name.
Variation: Aurore (Fr). See also Dawn, Roxane, Zarah.

Averil

Origin/meaning: Old English 'boar-battle'.
This name is now almost always feminine, despite its meaning, although it can be used for boys or girls. It is sometimes confused with Avril, the French form of April.
Variations: Averell, Averilla, Averyl, Everild, Everilda.

Avice (pron. Aviss)

Origin/meaning: Old German 'battle struggle'.
The original Old German name arrived in England at the time of the Conquest in the French form Havoise from which Avice derives.
Variations and abbreviations: Avicia, Avis. See also Hedwig.

Ayesha (pron. Ay'sha)

Origin/meaning: Arabic 'life' or 'alive'.
This popular Muslim name commemorates Ayesha, 610–677, the favorite of Mohammed's nine wives. He died on the 8th June, 632, with his head resting on her lap.
Variations: Aisha, Ashaas (Swahili), Ay'sha, Ayeshah.

Ayo

Origin/meaning: Yoruba 'joy'.
A Nigerian name. The word occurs in many other names such as Ayobami 'I am blessed with joy', Ayodele 'joy comes home', Ayoluwa 'joy of our people', Bayo 'joy is found', Dayo 'joy arrives', Nayo 'we have joy' and Olubayo 'highest joy'.

Aziza

Origin/meaning: Arabic 'precious'.
This is a common Muslim name.

Azra

Background: Arabic 'virgin'.

A long-established name given to of the mistress of Wamiq, a legendary lover who is found in Persian and Urdu poetry.

B

Babette

Origin/meaning: Hebrew 'God is my satisfaction'.

A short form of Elizabeth q.v. and occasionally of Barbara q.v.

Barbara

Origin/meaning: Greek 'stranger', 'foreigner'.

This was a popular medieval name in Europe given to girls in honor of a legendary St Barbara who was martyred by her own father.

Variations and abbreviations: Bab, Babbie (Scot), Babetta (It), Babette (Fr), Babita, Babs, Bar, Barbarina (It), Barb, Barbe (Fr), Barbie, Barbra (Dan), Barbro (Swed), Barby, St Barbe, Varina, Varinka, Varvara (Slav).

Bathsheba

Origin/meaning: Hebrew 'daughter of the oath' or 'voluptuous'.

King David sent Bathsheba's husband Uriah into the most dangerous area of battle so that he was killed. David was then able to marry her himself. Bathsheba became the mother of King Solomon.

Variations and abbreviations: Bathshua, Batsheva, Sheba.

Beatrice (pron. Béeatriss)

Origin/meaning: Latin 'bringer of happiness'.

This is the Italian form of the name given to honor St Beatrice, an early Roman martyr. Its revival in the 19th century was inspired by Dante's great poem 'The Divine Comedy'. In this he describes meeting his ideal love, Beatrice, in Paradise.

Variations and abbreviations: Bea, Beat, Beate, Béatrice (Fr), Beatricia, Beatrisa, Beatrix (Lat/Old Eng/Ger/Dut), Beatriz (Sp), Bee, Beitris (Scot), Bettrys (Wel), Bice (It), Biche (Fr), Trix, Trixi, Trixie, Trixy.

Beatrix

Origin/meaning: Latin 'bringer of happiness'.

Old (Latin) form of Beatrice q.v.

B

Girls' Names

Becky
Origin/meaning: Hebrew 'knotted cord' therefore 'faithful wife', or possibly 'heifer'.
A short form of Rebecca q.v.

Belinda
Origin/meaning: Old German 'snake-like', 'sinuous'.
The word 'linda' means snake. Snakes were regarded as magical or godlike by many communities including the Saxon peoples. This is therefore a complimentary name. It was used by Alexander Pope in his 'Rape of the Lock', 1712, and this gave it a certain currency.
Variations and abbreviations: Bel, Belle, Linda.

Belle
Origin/meaning: French 'beautiful'.
Also a short form of names such as Anabel, Arabella, Belinda, Isabel etc.
Variations and abbreviations: Anwen (Wel), Bell, Bella. See also Shobha.

Benita
Origin/meaning: Latin 'blessed'.
A Spanish feminine form of the masculine name Benedict.

Berenice
Origin/meaning: Greek 'bringer of victory'.
As a Biblical name, Berenice was the daughter of King Agrippa (Acts 25–26). The name is common in the US as Bernice.
Variations and abbreviations: Berenike (Ger), Bérénice (Fr), Berenice (It), Bernice, Bernie, Berny, Bunny.

Bernadette
Origin/meaning: Old German 'resolute as a bear'.
A French feminine form of Bernard q.v. Its great popularity in the 20th century particularly in Ireland and among Catholics, is almost entirely due to St Bernadette of Lourdes, 1844–1879.
See also Bernardine.

Bernardine
Origin/meaning: 'resolute as a bear'.
Rare feminine equivalent of Bernard q.v.
Variations and abbreviations: Berna, Bernadene, Bernadetta (It), Bernadette (Fr), Bernadina, Bernadine, Bernarda, Bernarde (Fr), Bernardina (It/Sp), Berneta, Bernie, Berny.

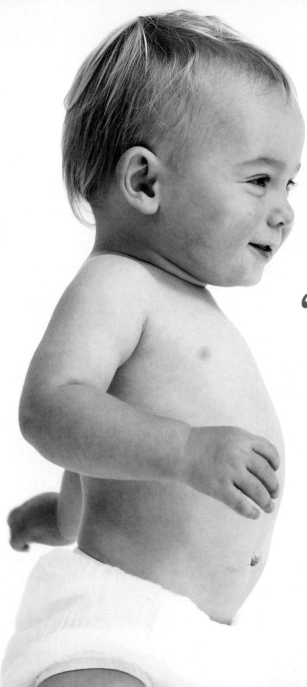

" The central struggle of parenthood is to let our hopes for our children outweigh our fears. **"**

Ellen Goodman

B

Girls' Names

Bertha

Origin/meaning: Old German 'bright'.

Bertha and Berta have been current in Europe since Saxon times. Because of its meaning the name was associated with the Feast of the Epiphany (January 6th) when the Magi followed the bright star to Bethlehem. So it became customary to give the name to girls born at that season.

Variations and abbreviations: Bert, Berta (Ger/It/Swed/Sp), Berte, Bertel (Ger), Berthe (Fr), Bertie, Bertina, Betty. See also Candida.

Beryl

Origin/meaning: Greek/Latin. A beryl is a precious stone, similar to an emerald, usually pale green, blue or white.

This is one of the precious stone names, which came into use in the 19th century at about the same time as flower names.

Variation: Berylla.

Bess

Origin/meaning: Hebrew 'God is my satisfaction'.

An English familiar form of Elizabeth q.v. often used for Elizabeth I who was popularly known as 'Good Queen Bess'.

Variations: Bessie, Bessy, Betsy.

Beth

Origin/meaning: Hebrew 'God is my satisfaction'.

English familiar form of Elizabeth q.v. sometimes used as an independent name.

Bethany

Origin/meaning: Aramaic 'house of poverty'.

A Biblical name (it was a small village near Jerusalem), this has been found from time to time in England and New England since the Reformation.

Bettina

Origin/meaning: Hebrew 'God is my satisfaction'.

An Italian short form of Elizabeth, popular in the 1960s, perhaps because of the famous model Bettina, wife of the Aly Khan.

Bettrys

Origin/meaning: Latin 'bringer of happiness'.

Welsh form of Beatrice q.v.

Variations: Beitiris (Scot Gaelic).

Betty

Origin/meaning: Hebrew 'God is my satisfaction'.

English familiar form of Elizabeth q.v. now often found as an independent name.
Variations: Beithidh (Gaelic), Betta (It), Bette, Betti (Ger), Bettie, Bettina (It), Betsey, Betsy. See also Elizabeth.

Beulah

Origin/meaning: Hebrew 'married', 'matronly'.
Variation: Beula.

Beverley

Origin/meaning: Old English 'from the beaver stream'.
A last name derived from a place in Yorkshire, this has since been used as a first name. The reason for its popularity in the US was originally the novel by G. B. McCutchan, 'Beverly of Graustark', 1904. The heroine was a Southern belle. The name is occasionally used for a boy.
Variations and abbreviations: Bev, Beverle, Beverlee, Beverly.

Bhavana (pron. Báunah)

Origin/meaning: Sanskrit 'conception', 'faith', 'love'.

Bianca

Origin/meaning: Italian 'white', 'fair'.
The Italian form of the French name Blanche q.v. Intended to imply fair in the sense of 'beautiful' as well as fair coloring as in Shakespeare's play 'The Taming of the Shrew'.
Variations: Biancamaria, Biancha (Med Eng), Bianka.

Billie

Origin/meaning: Old German 'helmet of resolution'.
A short form of feminine versions of William, e.g. Wilhelmina, Williamina. Sometimes given as an independent name.
Variations: Bill, Billee, Billi, Billy. See also Minnie.

Birgitta

Origin/meaning: Old Norse 'mountain stronghold' or Old Irish 'strong one'.
This is the Scandinavian form of Bridget q.v. The Swedish St Birgitta 1303–1373 was the wife of a nobleman and mother of eight children. She reformed the behavior and morals of the royal family.
Variations and abbreviations: Berget, Birga, Birgit, Brig, Brigga, Brigitta, Brita, Britt, Britta, Gita, Gitta.

Blanca

Origin/meaning: Spanish 'white', 'fair'.
Blanca of Castile married Louis VIII of France, and became the mother of Louis IX, St Louis. The French translated her name directly into their own language as Blanche.

Girls' Names

Blanche
Origin/meaning: French 'white' from Old German 'blaecan' to whiten.
A French name in its own right since the early Middle Ages, which was brought to England by the French wife of the Earl of Lancaster, a member of the royal family. It was one of the medieval names popularized in the 19th century.
Variations and abbreviations: Bianca (It), Blanca (Dan/Sp), Blanch, Blanchette (Fr), Blanchia, Blanka (Ger/Swed), Blaunch (Med Eng), Blinnie, Blinny. See also Arianwen, Blodwen, Candida, Guinevere.

Blodwen
Origin/meaning: Old Welsh 'white flower'.
Rare outside Wales.
Variation: Blodwyn.

Blossom
Origin/meaning: Old English 'flower-like'.
A flower name that became a popular given name, along with other flowers, in the 19th century.

Blythe
Origin/meaning: Old English 'gentle', 'cheerful'.
An unusual name, occasionally used as a boy's name.
Variations: Blithe, Blyth.

Bonita
Origin/meaning: Latin 'good', Spanish 'pretty'.
A Spanish name also used in the United States.
Variations and abbreviations: Bona (It), Bonnie, Nita.

Bonnie
Origin/meaning: Scots dialect 'pretty' perhaps derived from Latin bonus – good.
A name used as a familiar form of many names beginning with B and sometimes found as an independent name.
Variations: Bonnee, Bonni, Bonny.

Branwen
Origin/meaning: Old Welsh 'beautiful raven', 'raven-haired'.
Rare outside Wales. In the collection of old Welsh tales 'The Mabinogion', Branwen was the beautiful daughter of the British King Llyr, who married the King of Ireland.
Variations: Brangwain, Brengwain. See also Bronwen.

Bree

Origin/meaning: Irish 'hill'.

An old name that has become better known recently due to a character in the US TV series 'Desperate Housewives'.

Brenda

Origin/meaning: Old Norse 'sword'.

This name comes from the Shetland Isles off Scotland, which were settled by Viking invaders. It is the feminine form of Brand.

Briana

Origin/meaning: Old Irish 'strong'.

Modern feminine form of Brian q.v.

Variations: Brianne, Bryana.

Bridget

Origin/meaning: Old Irish 'strong one', 'mighty one' from the name of the Irish Celtic goddess of fire.

St Brigid of Kildare, 450–523, was the founder of the first convents in Ireland and she was greatly revered. For centuries Brigid and Mary have been the most popular female names in Ireland. Before the 17th century they were considered too sacred to be used. The usual form for a long time was Bride – or Bryde.

Variations and abbreviations: Bedelia, Beret, Berget, Biddie, Biddy, Birga, Birgit (Ger), Birgitta (Swed), Birte, Birtha, Brid (Ir), Bride, Bridie, Brietta, Brig, Brigga, Brighid (Ir), Brigid (Ir), Brigida (It/Sp), Briqide, Briqit (Ir), Brigitta (Swed/Ger), Brigitte (Fr/Ger), Brita, Britt (Swed), Britta (Swed), Bryde, Ffaod (Wel), Gita, Gitta.

Britt

Origin/meaning: Old Irish 'strong one', 'mighty one' or Old Norse 'mountain stronghold'.

A Swedish short form of Bridget q.v. from the form Brigitta.

Variations and abbreviations: Birte, Birtha, Brita, Britta. See Birgitta.

Bronwen

Origin/meaning: Old Welsh 'white breast'.

Common in Wales but rare elsewhere. It is a name which features in the collection of Welsh mythological tales 'The Mabinogion'.

Variations and abbreviations: Bron, Bronwyn.

Brooke

Origin/meaning: Old English 'brook'.

A common last name used as a first name, particularly in the US.

Variations: Brooks.

Brunhilda
Origin/meaning: Old German 'breast plate of battle', 'battle maid'.
The name of one of the Valkyrie, the twelve nymphs of Valhalla in ancient German and Norse legend. The name became known in English-speaking countries because of the popularity of Wagner's opera sequence 'The Ring of the Niebelung'.

Bryony
Origin/meaning: a climbing plant found in English hedgerows.

Buffy
Origin/meaning: Hebrew 'God is my satisfaction'.
A pet form of Elizabeth that has become known as a first name because of the TV series 'Buffy, the Vampire Slayer'.

Bunty
Origin/meaning: a term of endearment probably meaning plump or cuddly.
See also Bonnie.

C

Cadence
Origin/meaning: Latin 'rhythm'.
Variations: Cadena, Cadenza (Ital).

Caitlin
Origin/meaning: uncertain. Possibly Greek 'pure'.
An old Irish form of Kathleen.
Variation: Catlin (Eng), Kaitlin, Katelyn, Katlyn.

Callista
Origin/meaning: Greek 'most beautiful'.
Variations and abbreviations: Calesta, Calista, Callie, Calysta, Kalista.

Calypso
Origin/meaning: Greek 'concealer'.
In Greek myth Calypso was a nymph, Queen of the Isle of Ogygia (Gozo, near Malta) who kept Odysseus as her captive.

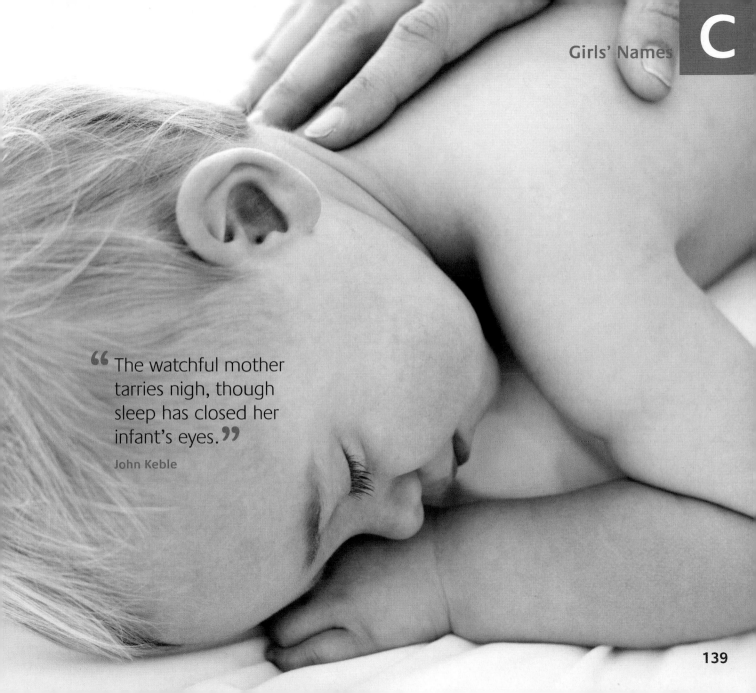

> "The watchful mother tarries nigh, though sleep has closed her infant's eyes."
>
> John Keble

Girls' Names

Camilla

Origin/meaning: Latin 'attendant at a sacrifice'.
Camilla was a female attendant. In the 18th-century classical revival Camilla became quite popular. Fanny Burney's novel 'Camilla', 1796, may have contributed to this.
Variations and abbreviations: Cam, Camila (Sp), Camille (Fr), Cammie, Kamilla (Ger), Millie, Milly.

Camille

Origin/meaning: Latin 'attendant at a sacrifice'.
The French version of the Latin/Italian name Camilla q.v.

Candace (pron. Cánndiss)

Origin/meaning: Greek 'glittering', 'bright white'.
One of many names which mean white. Candace was the name given to the Queens of Ethiopia.
Variations and abbreviations: Candi, Candice, Candie, Candy, Kandace, Kandy.

Candida

Origin/meaning: Latin 'white', 'fair', 'pure'.
The name was given some currency in the last century by George Bernard Shaw's play 'Candida', 1898.
Variations and abbreviations: Candi, Candide (Fr), Candy, Kandida (Ger).

Cara (pron. Cárr-a)

Origin/meaning: either Latin 'beloved' or Old Irish 'friend'.
Only becoming popular in the 20th century in English-speaking countries. The variation Kara is gaining popularity.
Variations: Carina (It), Carita (It), Carrie, Carry, Kara (US) (Kara is also pron. Care-uh).

Carla

Origin/meaning: Old German 'man', meaning by association 'womanly'.
An Italian feminine form of Charles q.v.

Carlotta

Origin/meaning: Old German 'man', meaning by association 'womanly'.
An Italian feminine form of Charles q.v.

Carly

Origin/meaning: Old German 'man', meaning by association 'womanly'.
A pet form of feminine versions of Charles. Used to be very popular because of singer Carly Simon. Celebrity Twiggy named her baby after her.
Variations: Carlie, Karlie, Karly.

Carmel

Origin/meaning: Hebrew 'garden'.

The name of the famous Mountain in Israel, Mount Carmel. The influential Order of Carmelite nuns drew their name from it, hence its use as a name for Catholic girls.

Variations and abbreviations: Carmela (It), Carmelina, Carmelita, Carmen (Sp), Carmencita, Carmina, Carmine, Carmita, Charmaine (Fr), Lita.

Carmen

Origin/meaning: Hebrew 'garden' or occasionally Latin 'song', 'poem'.

The Spanish form of Carmel q.v. The title of Bizet's opera.

Variations and abbreviations: Carma, Carmencita, Charmaine (Fr), Carmina.

Carol

Origin/meaning: Old German 'man', meaning by association 'womanly'. Sometimes given as Old French 'joyous song'.

A comparatively recent 20th-century name, Carol is connected to other feminine versions of Charles q.v. It may have begun as a shortened form of the 18th-century form Caroline.

Variations and abbreviations: Carola, Carole (Fr), Carroll, Carrie, Caryl, Carry, Karol, Karole, Karroll, Karoly.

Caroline

Origin/meaning: Old German 'man', meaning by association 'womanly'.

A feminine form of Charles introduced into England from Germany, when Caroline of Brandenburg-Anspach married the future George II. The form Carolyn is gaining popularity.

Variations and abbreviations: Carlin, Carlina, Carlyn, Carlynn, Caro, Carolin, Carolina (It/Sp), Carolyn, Carolynn, Carolynne, Carrie, Karoline (Ger), Karolyn, Lyn.

Casey

Origin/meaning: Greek 'unheeded prophetess'.

The popular boy's name derives from the 19th-century hero train driver of the 'Cannonball Express' who saved the lives of passengers at the expense of his own. However, as a girl's name it is considered to have started as a short form of Cassandra that then became a given name in its own right.

Cassandra

Origin/meaning: Greek, uncertain, possibly 'disbelieved by men'.

Cassandra was a Trojan prophetess and the sister of their hero Hector. Stories about the Trojan Wars were immensely popular in the Middle Ages and Cassandra became a fairly common name.

Variations and abbreviations: Casandra (Sp), Cass, Cassandre (Fr), Cassandry, Cassie, Cassy, Sandie, Sandy.

C

Girls' Names

Catharine/Catherine
Origin/meaning: uncertain; possibly Greek 'pure'.
A variant spelling of Katherine q.v.
Variations and abbreviations: Caitlin (Ir), Caitrin (It), Cass, Cassy, Catalina (Sp), Catarina (It), Cate, Caterina, Cath, Catharina, Catherina, Cathie, Cathleen (Ir), Cathlene, Cathrine, Cathryn, Cathy, Catie, Catriona (Scot). See also Katherine.

Catriona
Origin/meaning: uncertain, possibly Greek 'pure'.
Scottish form of Katharine q.v. Used by Robert Louis Stevenson as the title of one of his novels in 1893.
Variations and abbreviations: See Kathleen, Katharine.

Cecilia
Origin/meaning: Latin 'blind'.
Popular in the Middle Ages. St Cecilia was a martyr whose cult began in the 6th century and she became patron saint of music.
Variations and abbreviations: Caecilia, Celia, Cis.

Cecily (pron. Sissillee or Sessillee)
Origin/meaning: Latin 'blind'. From the Roman family Caecilius.
Introduced into Britain by William the Conqueror, who gave it to one of his daughters. It gave rise to several last names.
Variations and abbreviations: Cecil, Cécile (Fr), Cecilia, Celia, Cicely, Cissie, Cissy, Sheila, Shelagh (Ir), Sisley, Sissie, Sissy, Zazilie, Zilla.

Celeste
Origin/meaning: Latin 'heavenly'.
A French variation of Celia q.v.
Variations and abbreviations: Cele, Celesta, Celestia, Celestina (It), Celestine (Fr), Celestyn, Celestyna, Celina.

Celia
Origin/meaning: either 'heavenly' from the Ancient Roman family Caelius or 'blind' from the Ancient Roman family Caecilius.
The first meaning is probably correct. Celia is often assumed to be an abbreviated form of the quite distinct name Cecilia q.v.
Variations and abbreviations: Caelia, Celiana (It), Célie (Fr), Celeste (Fr), Celestine (Fr), Zilia.

Chandra (pron. Chandráh)
Origin/meaning: Sanskrit 'moon'.

Chantal (pron. Shontell)
Origin/meaning: A French place-name, Chantal or Cantal.
It honors St Jeanne Françoise de Chantal, 1572–1641, founder of a religious order.

Chardonnay

Origin/meaning: a white wine made from the grape of the same name.

First used as a given name when used as the name of a scheming female main character in the British TV drama series 'Footballers' Wives'.

Charis (pron. Káriss)

Origin/meaning: Greek 'grace', 'love'.

A 17th-century literary name. Also the origin of the word Charisma which means an ability to inspire devotion.

Variations and abbreviations: Carissa, Carrie, Charissa. See also Grace.

Charity

Origin/meaning: Greek 'grace', Latin 'affection', English 'charity', 'Christian love'.

One of the three virtues, spoken of by St Paul: 'And now abideth faith, hope, charity, these three; but the greatest of these is charity'. A name popular with the Puritans.

Variations and abbreviations: Carita (It), Caritina (It), Chattie, Cherry. See also Charis.

Charlene

Origin/meaning: Old German 'man', meaning by implication 'womanly'.

A feminine form of Charles popular in the US.

Variations: Carleen, Carlene, Carline, Charleen, Karleen, Karlene, Sharleen, Sharline.

Charlotte (pron. Shárlott)

Origin/meaning: Old German 'man', meaning by implication 'womanly'.

One of many feminine forms of Charles. In the 18th century it was used by the royal family, in particular Charlotte, wife of George III and Charlotte, Princess of Wales, daughter of George IV.

Variations and abbreviations: Carlota, Carlotta (It), Charleen, Charlene, Charlie, Charlotta, Chatty, Karlotta, Karlotte, Lola, Lolita, Lotta, Lotte, Lotti, Lottie, Tot, Tottie. See also Carla, Carol, Caroline and Cheryl.

Charmaine

Origin/meaning: Hebrew 'garden'.

The French form of the Irish Carmel and Spanish Carmen.

Chausiku (pron. Chaooséekoo)

Origin/meaning: Swahili 'born at night'.

Chere (pron. Shehr)

Origin/meaning: French 'dear', 'darling'.

A French adjective used mainly in North America as a given name.

Variations and abbreviations: Cher, Chérie (Fr), Chery, Cherry, Sher, Sherry.

Girls' Names

Cheryl
Origin/meaning: Old German 'man', usually given as 'womanly'.
Short form of Charlotte q.v.
Variations and abbreviations: Charil, Charyl, Cherlyn, Cherry, Sharyl, Sheryl.

Chipo
Origin/meaning: Shona 'gift'.
A Zimbabwe name.

Chiquita
Origin/meaning: Spanish 'little one'.
An endearment sometimes used as an independent name.

Chitra
Origin/meaning: Hindu 'picture'.

Chloë (pron. Klo-ee)
Origin/meaning: Greek 'a tender green shoot'.

Chris
Origin/meaning: Latin 'Christian' or 'Christ bearer'.
A short form of Christian, Christopher or Christine, sometimes used as an independent name.
Variations: Cris, Kris.

Christabel
Origin/meaning: Greek/Latin 'beautiful Christian'.
A Medieval English first name used by Samuel Taylor Coleridge as the title of one of his best-known poems, 'Christabel', 1816.
Variations and abbreviations: Chris, Christabell, Christabella, Christabelle, Christobel, Christobella, Christy.

Christiana
Origin/meaning: Latin 'Christian'.
Used as a Christian name since the early Middle Ages. It is related to the Scandinavian name Kirsten from which comes the Scottish name Kirsty.
Variations and abbreviations: Cairistiona (Scot), Chris, Christian, Christiania, Christiane (Fr), Cristiana (It), Cristiona (Ir), Kristyan.

Christine/Christina
Origin/meaning: Old English 'Christian'.
The English version was Latinized as Christina. St Christine was an early Christian martyr.

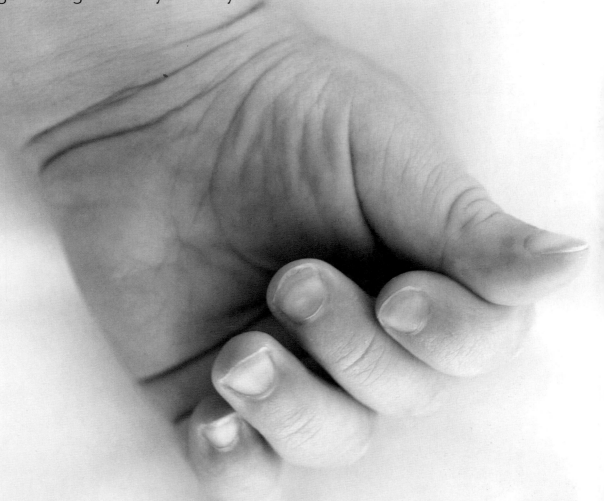

“Making the decision to have a child – it's momentous. It is to decide forever to have your heart go walking outside your body.”

Elizabeth Stone

C

Girls' Names

Variations and abbreviations: Chris, Chrissie, Chrissy, Christa, Christen, Christer, Christiana, Christie, Christin (Ger), Christy, Christyna, Cris, Crissie, Crissy, Cristie, Cristina (It/Sp), Cristine, Cristy, Kirsteen (Scot), Kirsten (Scand), Kirstyan, Kris, Krissie, Kristina, Krystyna, Tina.

Ciara
Origin/meaning: Old Irish 'dark haired'.
The feminine equivalent of the Irish masculine Kieran.
Variation: Ciaran.

Cindy
Origin/meaning: a pet form, particularly popular in the US, of names like Lucinda and Cynthia q.v.
Variation: Sindy.

Claire/Clare
Origin/meaning: Latin 'bright', 'distinguished'.
The veneration of St Clare of Assisi, 1193–1253, a friend of St Francis and founder of the Order of Nuns the Poor Clares, led to the name's increasing popularity. Appropriately, since the name is one of the most popular contemporary names, she is patron saint of television.
Variations: Chiara (It), Clair, Clara, Clarabelle, Claribel, Clarice, Clarie, Clarinda, Clarissa, Clarita (Sp), Clarrie, Klara (Ger), Klarissa.

Claudette
Origin/meaning: Latin 'lame'.
A French pet form of Claudia q.v.

Claudia
Origin/meaning: Latin 'lame'.
Used in England since the end of the 16th century, Claudia is mentioned in the second Epistle of St Paul to Timothy.
Variations: Claude (Fr), Claudette, Claudie, Claudina, Claudine, Gladys, Gwladys (Wel), Klaudia (Ger).

Clea
Origin/meaning: a name used by Lawrence Durrell in his novel sequence 'The Alexandria Quartet'. It may be a form of Clio q.v.

Clementine
Origin/meaning: Latin 'gentle', 'merciful'.
A feminine form of Clement.
Variations and abbreviations: Clementia, Clementina, Klementina.

Cleo
Origin/meaning: Greek 'fame', 'renown'.
A short form of Cleopatra which means 'renown of the father'.

Clio

Origin/meaning: Greek 'I celebrate', 'I proclaim'.
In Greek and Roman mythology Clio was the goddess of epic poetry and history.

Clodagh (pron. Clóh-duh)

Origin/meaning: Irish. It is the name of a river in Tipperary.
A 20th-century innovation, it rapidly became popular in Ireland.

Colette

Origin/meaning: Greek/Old French 'victory of the people'.
A diminutive of Nicolette. The French author, Colette, who wrote 'Gigi', boosted the name's popularity in the 20th century.
Variations: Colecta, Coletta, Collette.

Colleen

Origin/meaning: Old Irish 'girl'.

Connie

Origin/meaning: Latin 'constancy'.
A short form of Constance sometimes used as an independent name.

Constance

Origin/meaning: Latin 'constancy'.
The name of one of William I's daughters, it was introduced into England at the Conquest.
Variations and abbreviations: Con, Conni, Connie, Conny, Constancia, Constancy, Constantia, Constanze, Costanza (It), Konstanze (Ger).

Consuelo (pron. Konsooélla)

Origin/meaning: Spanish 'consolation'.
This is a short version of Our Lady of Consolation, a popular epithet of the Virgin Mary in Spain where it is Nuestra Señora del Consúelo.
Variations and abbreviations: Connie, Consolata, Consuela. See also Mercedes.

Coral

Origin/meaning: Greek 'red-pink coral'.
A name introduced at the end of the 19th century.
Variations: Coralie (Fr), Coraline.

C

Girls' Names

Cordelia
Origin/meaning: uncertain. Possibly Old Welsh 'jewel of the sea' or Latin 'warmhearted'.
The Latinized Celtic name Cordula may be the origin of the name Cordeilla, which Shakespeare adapted for the heroine of his play 'King Lear'.
Variations and abbreviations: Cordélie (Fr), Cordey, Cordie, Cordula, Cordy, Delia, Della, Kordela (Ger), Kordelia, Kordula.

Corinna
Origin/meaning: Greek, from the word 'maiden'.
An ancient Greek name sometimes used for the goddess of Spring, Persephone.
Variations: Corena, Corene, Corina, Corinne (Fr).

Cornelia
Origin/meaning: Latin, from the influential Roman family Cornelius. The name may be from 'horn' which implies kingship.
The feminine form of Cornelius q.v. It was the name of Julius Caesar's first wife.
Variations and abbreviations: Cornela, Cornelie (Fr), Cornie, Corry, Kornelia (Ger), Nelia, Nell, Nelly.

Cosima
Origin/meaning: Greek 'order', 'harmony', 'the universe'.
Italian feminine form of Cosmo q.v.
Variation: Kosima (Ger).

Courtney
Origin/meaning: either Old French 'short nose' or de Courtenay, an aristocratic family from Courtenay in France.
The family name of the West Country Earls of Devon. It was particularly successful in the US.
Variations and abbreviations: Court, Courtnay, Curt.

Cressida
Origin/meaning: Greek 'daughter of the golden one'.
The name Crysëis was wrongly used by Boccacio for the faithless daughter of Calchas. He adapted the name slightly to Chryseida and Chaucer altered it further to Criseyde. When Shakespeare wrote 'Troilus and Cressida' he altered the name once more.
Abbreviation: Cressy.

Crystal
Origin/meaning: Greek 'clear-ice', 'crystal'.
A modern girl's name dating from the end of the 19th century
Variations: Chrystal, Krystle.

Cynthia

Origin/meaning: Greek 'from Mount Cynthia'.
A title used for Artemis, the Greek goddess of chastity and hunting, who was born on Mount Cynthos.
Variations and abbreviations: Cimmie, Cindee, Cindie, Cindy, Cynthie. See also Phoebe.

D

Dagmar

Origin/meaning: Old German 'glory of the Danes'.
A Danish name. The Empress Dagmar of Russia was a sister of Queen Alexandra.

Daisy

Origin/meaning: Old English 'day's eye'. The name of a flower.
A late 19th-century name. Sometimes it was used as a pet name for Margaret, since its French equivalent, Marguerite, is the French word for a daisy.

Damayanti

Origin/meaning: Sanskrit 'subduing (men by beauty)'.
In Hindu legend, the name of a beautiful princess whose courtship with her husband, Prince Nala, was carried out by the mediation of swans.

Dana (pron. Day-nuh)

Origin/meaning: uncertain, possibly Scandinavian 'Danish'.

Danielle

Origin/meaning: Hebrew 'God has judged'.
French feminine form of Daniel q.v.
Variations and abbreviations: Danella, Danelle, Danette, Daniela (It/Sp), Darnella, Dannie, Danny.

Daphne

Origin/meaning: Greek 'laurel bush', 'bay tree'.
Daphne in Greek mythology was a nymph loved by Apollo. She called on the gods to help her elude his advances and they obliged by turning her into a laurel bush. The name came into use as a girl's name at the end of the 19th century.
Variations and abbreviations: Dafne, Daffie, Daph.

Girls' Names

Darcy

Origin/meaning: Old French 'from Arcy', Old Irish 'dark man'.
This is a name that came to England as a last name with William the Conqueror. It became an Irish first name after a branch of the family settled there in the late Middle Ages.
Variations and abbreviations: D'Arcy, Darsey, Darsy.

Darlene

Origin/meaning: Old English 'darling'.
Modern feminine version of the much older established masculine name Daryl q.v. Found mainly in North America.
Variations and abbreviations: Darla, Darleen, Darelle, Daryl, Darylyne.

Davina

Origin/meaning: Hebrew 'darling', 'friend'.
A Scottish feminine form of David. Dating from the 17th century.
Variations and abbreviations: Davida (Eng), Davidina, Davinia, Davita, Veda, Vida, Vita.

Dawn

Origin/meaning: English 'sunrise'.
A modern 20th-century innovation. There are many names of differing origins with the same meaning including Aurora, Zara, Roxanne and Oriana.

Deborah

Origin/meaning: Hebrew 'bee'.
Deborah was a Jewish prophetess (Judges 5). The name's great popularity in the 20th century is perhaps because of the influence of film stars such as Debbie Reynolds and Deborah Kerr.
Variations and abbreviations: Deb, Debor, Debora, Debra, Debbie, Debby. See also Melissa.

Deirdre

Origin/meaning: Old Irish 'sorrowful' or 'raging'.
Deirdre was the tragic heroine of a Celtic legend, in which she committed suicide following the death of her lover and his brothers. W. B. Yeats wrote 'Deirdre' in 1907 and J. M. Synge wrote 'Deirdre of the Sorrows' in 1910, both based on the same legend.
Variations and abbreviations: Dede, Dee, Deerdre, Didi.

Delia

Origin/meaning: Greek 'from Delos'.
Delia is one of the names given to the Greek goddess Artemis, in this case because she came from the island of Delos. It may sometimes be used as a short form of Cordelia q.v.
Variations and abbreviations: Dee, Della, Didi.

"At a child's birth, if a mother could ask a fairy godmother to endow it with the most useful gift, that gift would be curiosity."

Eleanor Roosevelt

Girls' Names

Delilah
Origin/meaning: Hebrew 'delight'.
A Biblical name. Delilah betrayed Samson to the Philistines by cutting off the hair from which he derived his great strength (Judges 13–16).

Della
Origin/meaning: Old German 'noble'.
Familiar form of names such as Adèle and Delia, sometimes used as an independent name, particularly in North America.

Delmar
Origin/meaning: Spanish 'of the sea'.
Found in the US and Australia.
Variation: Delma.

Delphine
Origin/meaning: either Greek 'from Delphi' or Greek 'Delphinium' (a plant with a nectary resembling a dolphin). Delphine is the French version.
Variations and abbreviations: Delfa, Delpha, Delfina (It/Sp), Delfine (Ger), Delphina.

Denise
Origin/meaning: Greek, from the name of the god of fertility Dionysus.
French feminine version of Dennis.
Variations and abbreviations: Denice, Deniece, Denis, Denny, Denyse, Dion, Dionne.

Désirée (pron. Dáyzeeray)
Origin/meaning: Latin/French 'desired', 'longed for'.
This name arrived from France in the 20th century.
Variations: Desiderata, Desideria (Ger), Desire.

Devi
Origin/meaning: Sanskrit 'goddess'.
The feminine form of Dev that in Hindu texts is used to refer to the wife of Shiva.

Diana
Origin/meaning: Latin 'divine'. The Roman equivalent of Artemis, the Greek goddess of chastity, hunting and the moon.
The classical name came into use in Europe in the 16th and 17th centuries. Shakespeare used it in his play 'All's Well That Ends Well', written at the beginning of the 17th century.
Variations and abbreviations: Deana, Deanna, Dede, Dee, Di, Diane (Fr), Dianna, Dianora (It), Didi, Dyana, Dyanna.

Dido
Origin/meaning: obscure, possibly Greek 'teacher'.
Dido was the legendary founder and Queen of Carthage. In the poem by the Roman Virgil, he describes how she falls in love with Aeneas and kills herself when the gods order him to leave her.

Dilys
Origin/meaning: Welsh 'perfect' or 'pure'.
A recent Welsh name used in the last hundred years.

Dinah
Origin/meaning: Hebrew 'lawsuit' therefore 'avenged'.
In Genesis ch.34, Dinah is the daughter of Leah and Jacob. When she is dishonored by Shechem her brothers avenge her.
Variations and abbreviations: Dena, Di, Dina.

Dionne
Origin/meaning: Greek 'follower of Dionysus'.
A modern version of Denise q.v. found particularly in the US.
Variations: Dion, Dione, Dionis.

Divina
Origin/meaning: Latin 'divine' or 'super-human'.
A Latin adjective occasionally used as a first name.

Dolly
Origin/meaning: Greek 'gift of God'.
A short form of Dorothy q.v. which had been used as an independent name since the Middle Ages. It was so popular that in the 18th century it became the word which we still use today for toy babies.
Variations and abbreviations: Dol, Doll, Dollie.

Dominique
Origin/meaning: Latin 'of the Lord'.
French feminine form of Dominic q.v. equivalent of the Medieval English Dominica. It is sometimes used for a child born on Sunday, the Lord's day.

Donatella
Origin/meaning: Latin 'given'.
A pet form of Donata that is in turn a feminine form of Donato, a popular Renaissance name. Donatella is most famous for being the name of the fashion designer Donatella Versace, the sister of Gianni Versace, who took over the business when her brother was shot dead outside his Miami home in 1997.

D

Girls' Names

Dora
Origin/meaning: Greek 'gift'.
A short form of Dorothy or Theodora q.v. it became popular as a name in its own right at the end of the 19th century.
Variations and abbreviations: Dodie, Doralyn, Dorelle, Dorena, Doretta, Dorja (Russ), Dorrie, Doro, Dory.

Doreen
Origin/meaning: uncertain, either Old Irish 'sullen' or an Irish diminutive of Dorothy 'gift of God'.
Introduced into England from Ireland around the turn of the century.
Variations and abbreviations: Dora, Dorene, Dorine.

Doris
Origin/meaning: Greek 'gift'.
The name of a nymph in Greek mythology and the name of a small independent country in Ancient Greece. It came into use in the 19th century. Despite its apparent classical origins it is also likely to be a variation of the once popular Dorothy q.v.
Variations and abbreviations: Dorice, Dorise, Dorita, Dorris, Dory.

Dorothy
Origin/meaning: Greek 'gift of God'.
A back-to-front version of Theodora q.v. which has the same meaning. The name was not found in England until the 16th century. At the end of the 18th century the Latinized Dorothea became fashionable. The Scottish/Irish short form Dorrit, Dickens used for his novel 'Little Dorrit', 1857.
Variations and abbreviations: Darja (Russ), Dody, Doll, Dollie, Dolly, Dora, Doreen (Ir), Dorinda, Dorofeja (Russ), Doro, Dorotea (It/Sp), Dorothea (Ger), Dorothée (Fr), Dorrit (Ir), Dortea (Dan), Dorthea (Dan), Dorthy, Dory, Dot, Dottie, Dotty.

Drew
Origin/meaning: Old German 'bearer' or Old French 'vigorous'.
This is the Medieval English form of the name Drogo, by way of the French form Dru. Drogo lost its popularity after the 17th century but Drew survives, in the US particularly.
Variations: Drogo, Dru.

Dulcie
Origin/meaning: Latin 'sweet'.
Since the Middle Ages there have been names derived from dulcis, the Latin word meaning sweet. They include Dulcia and Dulcibelle, a typical 18th-century variation. Dulcie is the modern form found since the end of the 19th century.
Variations and abbreviations: Delcine, Dulce, Dulcea, Dulcia, Dulciana, Dulcibelle, Dulcine, Dulcinea, Dulcy.

Dusty
Origin/meaning: Old German 'brave warrior'.
Known as a boy's name until the 1960s when it was made popular as a feminine name by the singer Dusty Springfield.

E

Edie
Origin/meaning: Old English 'rich war'.
A form of Edith that has become fashionable as a given name in recent times.

Ebony
Origin/meaning: a name that derives from the shiny black wood.

Edina
Origin/meaning: Old English 'rich friend'.
This is a Scottish variation of Edwina, the feminine form of Edwin q.v.

Edith
Origin/meaning: Old English 'rich war'.
This is the modern form of the Anglo-Saxon name Eadgyth. The name was borne by several saints. One, St Edith (Eadgyth) of Wilton, 961–989, was an illegitimate daughter of King Edgar. The Normans changed Eadgyth to Eaditha, a common name in the Middle Ages.
Variations and abbreviations: Eaditha (Med Eng), Eda, Ede, Edie, Edita (It), Editha, Edithe, Edwa, Edyth, Eyde, Eydie.

Edna
Origin/meaning: uncertain, Hebrew 'rejuvenation'.
A Biblical name which occurs several times in the Apocrypha. In the Book of Tobia Edna is the mother of Sara and mother-in-law of Tobia.
Variations and abbreviations: Ed, Eddie, Ednah.

Edwina
Origin/meaning: Old English 'rich friend'.
A 19th-century feminine form of Edwin q.v.
Variations: Edina (Scot), Edwine.

Effie
Origin/meaning: Greek 'fair speech', implying either 'silence' or 'honor'.
A short form of Euphemia. Used in the 19th century particularly in Scotland.

Girls' Names

Eileen (pron. Eyeleen or Evleen)
Origin/meaning: Greek 'light' or 'bright' or Old Irish 'pleasant'.
This name is often used in Ireland as the Irish equivalent of Helen q.v. However the alternative pronunciation indicates that it is sometimes a version of Eveline, in which case it takes on the second meaning.
Variations and abbreviations: Aileen, Eily, Eveline.

Eirwen
Origin/meaning: Welsh 'white snow'.
A modern name with an ancient feel.

Eithne
Origin/meaning: Old Irish 'little fire', 'little fiery one'.
The modern spelling of the Old Irish name Aithne q.v.
Variation: Ethne. See also Ena.

Elaine
Origin/meaning: Greek 'light' or 'bright'.
The Medieval French form of the Greek name Helen q.v. The name was used in medieval literature and in particular the legends surrounding King Arthur and his Knights of the Round Table, which tell of Princess Elaine's doomed love for Sir Lancelot. This made the name a favourite among the Victorians.
Variations: Elain, Elana, Elane, Elayne.

Eleanor
Origin/meaning: Greek 'bright', 'light'.
Again this is a Medieval French form of the Greek name Helen q.v. It was introduced into England on the marriage of Eleanor of Aquitaine (1122–1204) with Henry II. The name gained popularity because of Edward I's much loved queen, Eleanor of Castile. On her death in 1290 he erected the famous stone crosses which marked the resting places of her body on its journey to London for burial.
Variations and abbreviations: Alienore, Eleanora, Eléanore (Fr), Elenore, Eleonore (It), Elianora, Elinor, Elinore, Ella, Ellie, Elly, Leonor (Sp), Lenore, Leonora, Leonore, Nell, Nellie, Nelly, Nora.

Elfrida
Origin/meaning: Old English 'elf-strength'.
A pre-Conquest Anglo-Saxon name.
Variations and abbreviations: Elfreda, Elfrid, Freda.

Eliana
Origin/meaning: Greek 'sun'.
This is an Italian name occasionally used in English-speaking countries. It is sometimes considered a feminine form of Elias/Elijah q.v.

"Whenever I held my newborn baby in my arms, I used to think that what I said and did to him could have an influence not only on him but on all whom he met, not only for a day or a month or a year, but for all eternity – a very challenging and exciting thought for a mother."

Rose Kennedy

E

Girls' Names

Elise
Origin/meaning: Hebrew 'God is my satisfaction'.
A French short form of Elizabeth now used as an independent name.
Variation: Elyse.

Eliza
Origin/meaning: Hebrew 'God is my satisfaction'.
A short form of Elizabeth. Used as a pet name for Elizabeth I in the 16th century. Shaw chose it for the heroine of his play 'Pygmalion' which was adapted as the musical 'My Fair Lady'.
Variations and abbreviations: Lisa, Liza, Elisa, Elise (Fr). See also Elizabeth.

Elizabeth
Origin/meaning: Hebrew 'God is my satisfaction'.
This is the usual English spelling of the name. It comes via the Latin spelling whereas the continental spelling, using 's' instead of 'z', comes directly from the Greek. It is Biblical, being the name of the mother of John the Baptist and the wife of Aaron. However in the 16th century the long and successful reign of Elizabeth I, 1533–1603, the daughter of Henry VIII and Anne Boleyn, brought the name from comparative obscurity to the point where nearly one girl in four was baptized Elizabeth. At different times different variations have found favor. For example, Bess in the 16th century, Betty in the 18th century and again in the mid-20th century, Eliza at the end of the 18th century and the 19th century. Lisa and Liza are fashionable at the moment.
Variations and abbreviations: Babette (Fr), Belita (Sp), Belle, Bess, Bessie, Bessy, Beth, Betsey, Betsy, Betta, Bette, Betti, Bettie, Bettina (It), Bettine (Fr), Betty, Ealasaid (Scot Gaelic), Eilis (Ir), Elisa (It), Elisabet (Scand), Elisabeth, Elisabetta (It), Elise (Fr), Elissa (It), Eliza, Elizabella, Elizabet, Elly, Elsa (Ger/Dut/Scand), Elsbeth (Scot), Else (Ger/Dut/Scand), Elsey, Elsie (Scot), Elspet (Scot), Elspeth (Scot), Elsy, Elyse, Helsa, Isabel, Isabella (Sp/It), Isabetta (It), Isobel (Scot), Lib, Libbie, Libby, Liesel (Ger), Lieschen (Ger), Lillibet, Lisa, Lisabeth, Lisavetta (Slav), Lisbeth, Lise (Ger), Liselotte (Ger), Lisette (Fr), Lissa, Liz, Liza, Lizabeth, Lizbeth, Lizzie, Lizzy, Ysabel (and see Isabel).

Ella
Origin/meaning: uncertain, probably Old German 'all'.
A popular medieval name brought to England by the Normans. In the US it was frequently used in compound names such as Ella-Jane and Ella-May.
Variations: Ellaline, Ellie, Elly.

Ellen
Origin/meaning: Greek 'light' or 'bright'.
This is the form of Helen used in medieval England and pre-Conquest Scotland and Wales. It was revived in the 19th century.
Variations and abbreviations: Ella, Ellie, Ellin, Ellyn.

Eloïse (pron. Elloweeze)

Origin/meaning: Old German 'flourishing and strong'.
The Normans adopted the name and brought it to England in the form of Helewis. In the 19th century when medieval themes were popular, the story of the doomed love of the 12th-century monk Abelard for his pupil Héloïse, revived interest in the name.
Variations: Eloisa (It), Helewise (Med Eng), Héloïse (Fr).

Elsa

Origin/meaning: Old German 'noble' or Hebrew 'God is my satisfaction'.
This predominantly German name was introduced to English-speaking countries in the 19th century when Wagner used it for the heroine of his opera 'Lohengrin', 1848.
Variations: Else, Ilsa, Ilse. See also Elizabeth.

Elspeth

Origin/meaning: Hebrew 'God is my satisfaction'.
An almost exclusively Scottish variation of Elizabeth.
Variations and abbreviations: Eilasaid, Elsbeth, Elsie, Elspet, Elspie.

Eluned (pron. Éllinedd)

Origin/meaning: uncertain. Possibly a reference to the Old Welsh word meaning 'idol'.
A popular Welsh name occasionally used in England. Its short form Lyn and the Medieval French form Lynnet have proved more popular in English-speaking countries than the original.
Variations and abbreviations: Eiluned, Elined, Linet, Luned, Lyn, Lynn, Lynnet, Lynette.

Elvira

Origin/meaning: uncertain, possibly Old German 'elf-counsel' or 'elf-ruler'.
This is a Spanish name which is found several times in literature, most notably as the woman seduced by Don Juan and as the heroine of Verdi's opera 'Ernani'. Made famous in US in the 80s & 90s by the TV and film personality 'Elvira: Mistress of the Dark'.
Variation: Elvire (Fr).

Emily

Origin/meaning: Latin, from the Roman clan name Aemelius.
This is a Medieval Italian name popularized by the Italian Renaissance poet Boccaccio. He used it in 'Il Teseide', which was read throughout Europe. Chaucer in 'The Knight's Tale' (1380) borrowed both the plot and the name from Boccaccio's story. Shakespeare used Emilia for Iago's wife in his play 'Othello'.
Variations and abbreviations: Amalia, Aimil (Scot), Em (Med Eng), Emalia, Emelye, Emerlee, Emilia (It/Sp), Emilie (Ger), Émilie (Fr), Emmie, Emmy.

Girls' Names

Emma

Origin/meaning: Old German 'universal' or from the name of the Teutonic god-hero Irmin.

This name probably began as a short form of names like Ermintrude and Ermendard. It was adopted by the Normans and in 1002 Emma, daughter of Richard I, Duke of Normandy, brought it to England when she married Ethelred the Unready. In 1016 after being widowed she married his successor, King Canute. Queen Emma was a popular figure and the name has been used ever since.

Variations and abbreviations: Em, Emm, Emmie, Emmot, Erma (Ger), Imma, Irma (Ger).

Emmanuelle

Origin/meaning: Hebrew 'God with us'.

Feminine form of Emanuel q.v.

Emmeline

Origin/meaning: Old German 'little industrious one'.

This is a diminutive of Amalburga, the original form of Amelia q.v. and introduced to England by the Normans. It was revived as part of the Romantic Movement's interest in medieval culture at the beginning of the 19th century.

Variations and abbreviations: Amelia, Em, Emblem, Emblin, Emelia, Emlin, Emlyn, Emmaline, Emmy.

Ena

Origin/meaning: Old Irish 'little fire' or 'little fiery one'.

This is an English form of the Celtic name Aine (pron. Awnye) who was Queen of the Fairies. Although generally considered Irish the name is increasingly found in Scotland.

Enid

Origin/meaning: uncertain, possibly Welsh 'tree-bark'.

This is another of the names, probably Welsh in origin, which have become more widely familiar through the tales of King Arthur and his Knights. Enid was the wife of Sir Geraint q.v. and wrongly considered by him to be unfaithful. However her selfless nursing when he was wounded convinced him he was mistaken and they lived happily ever after. Enid's virtues have sometimes led to the meaning of the name being given as 'purity'.

Erica

Origin/meaning: Old Norse 'ever-ruling'.

This is the feminine form of Eric q.v. Although popular for over 1000 years in Scandinavia it was not used in England until the 19th century. Erica was sometimes assumed to be a flower name since it is the Latin name for heather.

Variations and abbreviations: Eri, Ericha, Erika (Ger/Scand), Rickie, Rikkie.

Erin

Origin/meaning: Old Irish 'peace'.

This is an alternative Celtic name for Ireland. Its use as a personal name is modern.

Variations: Erina, Erinna.

Ermintrude

Origin/meaning: Old German 'universal strength' or 'strength of Irmin'. Irmin was one of the god-heroes like Ing.
A pre-Conquest name, it was revived in the early 19th century during the period of interest in early history.
Variations and abbreviations: Ermentrude, Ermyntrude, Irmintrude, Trudie, Trudy.

Esmé

Origin/meaning: French/Latin 'loved'.
This is a variation of Amy q.v. introduced from France to Scotland in the 16th century. It was originally a boy's name but by the time it spread to England it was also used for girls and is now considered primarily a girl's name. Esmé may also be a short form of the Spanish name Esmeralda.
Variations: see Amy.

Esmeralda

Origin/meaning: Spanish 'emerald'.
An extremely popular Spanish name. Its use by the Romantic writer Victor Hugo in his novel 'The Hunchback of Notre Dame', 1831, and the opera 'La Esmeralda', 1837, made the name familiar.
Variations and abbreviations: Emerald, Esmé, Esmeraldah.

Esperanza

Origin/meaning: Latin 'hope'
A name popular in Spain and now the US.

Estelle

Origin/meaning: Latin 'star'.
This is a French form of the name Stella. Occasionally used in English-speaking countries since Dickens gave Estella to a character in his novel 'Great Expectations', 1861.
Variations and abbreviations: see Stella.

Esther

Origin/meaning: uncertain. Probably Persian 'myrtle' or 'star'.
In the book of the Old Testament which carries her name, Esther is a Jewess who is chosen by King Ahasueras for her great beauty. Among non-Jewish people the name came into use in the 17th century. The play 'Esther', 1689, written by the French playwright Racine, may have given the name extra publicity.
Variations and abbreviations: Essa, Essie, Essy, Esta, Ester (It), Ettie, Etty, Hadassah, Hester, Hesther, Hettie, Hetty.

Ethel

Origin/meaning: Old English 'noble'.
This is a simplification of Aethel. The prefix Ethel was not used on its own in pre-Conquest times but always as part of the compound names such as Ethelred or Ethelfleda. In the 19th century, Ethel developed as an obvious short form. It was used in

Girls' Names

Thackeray's 'The Newcomes', 1855, which undoubtedly helped to establish it. The popularity of the Romantic novelist Ethel M. Dell, 1881–1939, may have influenced many mothers to choose the name during the period between the two World Wars.
Variations and abbreviations: Eth, Ethyl.

Eugenia
Origin/meaning: Greek 'noble', 'well-born'.
The Italian feminine form of Eugene. The stylish wife of the French Emperor Napoleon III, the Empress Eugénie, 1826–1920, created a fashion for the French form of the name in the 19th century.
Variations and abbreviations: Eugénie (Fr), Gene, Genia, Ginny.

Eva
Origin/meaning: uncertain. Possibly Hebrew 'life-giving'.
The Latinized form of Eve q.v. In English-speaking countries it was used increasingly after the publication of Harriet Beecher Stowe's book 'Uncle Tom's Cabin', 1852, which had the popular character 'little Eva'.

Evangeline
Origin/meaning: Greek 'brings good news'.
Became familiar after Henry Wadsworth Longfellow used it for his 1848 poem 'Evangeline' whose heroine is Evangeline Bellefontaine.

Eve
Origin/meaning: uncertain. Possibly Hebrew 'life-giving'.
This is the name given to the first woman by Adam.
Variations: Eva, Evie, Evita (Sp).

Eveline/Evelyn (pron. Ehv-linn in US)
Origin/meaning: Old French 'hazel-tree' or Old Celtic 'pleasant'.
The variation Evelyn, which is now more popular than the original spelling, is probably copied from the masculine Evelyn, q.v.
Variations: Avelina, Aveline, Avelyn, Eveleen, Evelina, Evelyn.

F

Fabia (pron. Fáybea)
Origin/meaning: Latin: of the Roman Fabius family.
This name is the root form of the diminutives Fabiana and Fabiola.

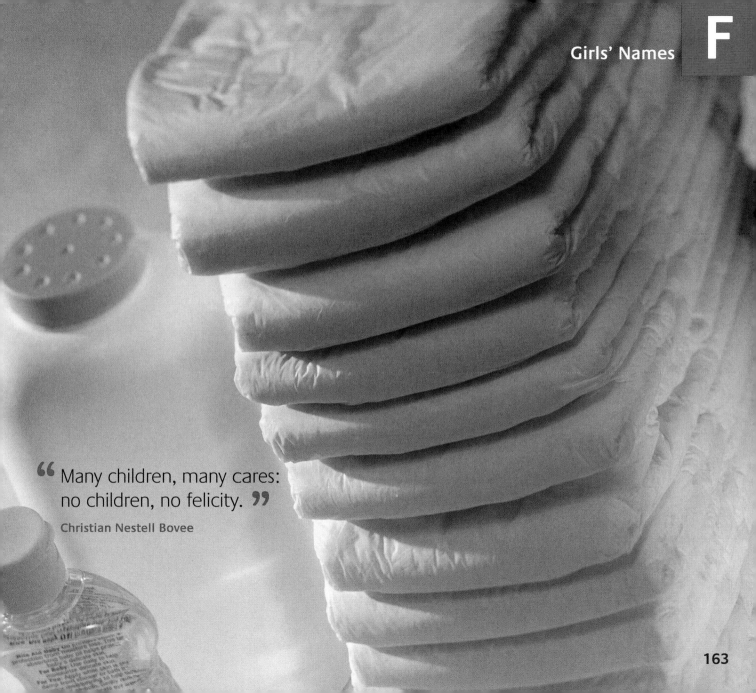

"Many children, many cares:
no children, no felicity."

Christian Nestell Bovee

Girls' Names

Fahmida
Origin/meaning: Arabic 'learned man'.
The Urdu feminine form of Fahim.
Variation: Fizza

Faith
Origin/meaning: Latin 'trust', 'faith'.
This, with Hope and Charity, was one of the three virtues referred to by St Paul in his first Epistle to the Corinthians.
Abbreviation: Fay.

Fanny
Origin/meaning: Late Latin 'free' or 'from France'.
A familiar form of Frances q.v. Used since the 18th century as an independent name.
Variation and abbreviation: see Frances.

Fatima (pron. Fáhteema)
Origin/meaning: Arabic 'daughter of the prophet' or 'weaned'.
Fatima was the youngest daughter of the Prophet Mohammed. She married Ali q.v. the first convert to Mohammedanism. There is also a similar Swahili name Fatuma (weaned) used for Fatima in parts of Africa.

Fay
Origin/meaning: either 'fairy' or an abbreviation of Faith q.v.
Like May, which may be the month or an abbreviation of Mary, Fay is a name which originated in the 19th century.
Variations: Fayanne, Faye, Fayette (Fr).

Felicia
Origin/meaning: Latin 'fortunate'.
This is a feminine form of Felix. It was popular in the Middle Ages when it was probably given to honor St Felicia, one of the many early martyrs.
Variations and abbreviations: Felice, Felicity, Felis, Félise (Fr), Phelisia.

Felicity
Origin/meaning: Latin 'happiness'.
This virtue name was adopted by 17th-century Puritans in preference to the saint's name Felicia.
Variations and abbreviations: Fee, Felicia, Félicité (Fr), Felicidad (Sp), Felicita (It), Felicissima (It), Felizia (Ger).

Fern
Origin/meaning: Sanskrit 'feather'.
This is the name of a woodland plant renowned for its feathery fronds. Ferns were popular houseplants in Victorian times and it is

not surprising that Fern should have come into use at the end of the 19th century when flower names were fashionable. Fern is sometimes found as a short form of the Italian name Fernanda.

Ffion (pron. Feeon)
Origin/meaning: Welsh 'roses'.
This is the Welsh equivalent of Rose or Rosanna.

Fidda
Origin/meaning: Arabic 'silver'.
A name that is particularly popular in Jordan.

Finola
Origin/meaning: Old Irish 'white shoulders'.
A modern Irish form of Fenella.

Fiona (pron. Feeówna)
Origin/meaning: Old Irish 'fair'.
This is a pen-name invented by the Scottish novelist William Sharp, 1855–1905. As Fiona Macleod, he wrote a series of novels inspired by the Old Celtic myths and legends. The name is now well established and has become increasingly popular since the Second World War.
Variations: Ffiona (Wel), Fionna.

Flavia (pron. Fláyvia)
Origin/meaning: Latin: from the Flavius family.
This was a well-known Roman name and is thought to be derived from the word flavus – yellow.
Variations: Flaviana, Flavilla.

Fleur
Origin/meaning: French 'flower'.
This is a modern equivalent of the classical name Flora q.v.
Variations: Fflyr (Wel), Flora, Florence, Flore (Med Fr), Flower.

Flora
Origin/meaning: Latin. The name of the Roman goddess of flowers and spring, and lover of the West Wind, Zephyr. Her festival was called the Floralia.
This name was used from time to time in the Middle Ages because of St Flora, martyred at Cordova in 851.
Variations and abbreviations: Fflyr (Wel), Fleur (Fr), Fleurette (Fr), Floella, Flor, Flore (Fr/Scot), Florella, Floretta, Floria, Floriane, Floris, Florrie. See also Fleur, Flower, Kusum.

F

Girls' Names

Florence
Origin/meaning: Latin 'in bloom' or 'prosperous'.
This name, often in the Latin form of Florentia, was used in England in the Middle Ages. There was also a masculine form, Florentius.
Variations and abbreviations: Fiorenza (Ir), Flo, Flora, Florance, Flore, Florencia (Sp), Florentina, Florenza (It), Florentia (Ger), Florenzia (Ger), Florenzina, Floria, Florie, Florina, Florinda, Floris, Florrie, Florry, Flossie, Flossy.

Flossie
Origin/meaning: Latin 'in bloom' or 'prosperous'.
A familiar form of Florence q.v. which was sometimes used at the end of the 19th century when Florence was a vogue name.
Variations and abbreviations: see Florence.

Flower
Origin/meaning: 'a flower'.
This word, like the French Fleur, has occasionally been used as a first name. However it is rare. The long-established Latin name Flora is usually preferred.

Folukè (pron. Folóokee)
Origin/meaning: Yoruba 'placed in God's care'.
This name comes from Nigeria.

Fran
Origin/meaning: Old German 'a Frank', Medieval Latin 'from France'.
A short form of Frances q.v. sometimes used as an independent name.
Variations: see Frances.

Frances
Origin/meaning: Medieval Latin 'from France' or 'free', both meanings from old German 'a Frank'.
This is the feminine form of the masculine name Francis q.v. Like Francis it was introduced to England in the Tudor period.
Variations and abbreviations: Fan, Fanchette (Fr), Fanchon (Fr), Fancy (US), Fannie, Fanny, Fran, Francelia, Francesca (It), Francesse, Francine, Francisca (Sp/Port), Francoise (Fr), Francyne, Frangag (Wel), Frank, Frankie, Frannie, Franny, Franziska (Ger), Frasquita (Sp), Zissi.

Francesca (pron. Franchéska)
Origin/meaning: Medieval Latin 'from France'.
This is the Italian form of Frances q.v. It is the earliest form of the name although a name of similar origin, Franka, predates it.
Variations and abbreviations: see Frances.

Françoise (pron. Frónswahze)

Origin/meaning: Medieval Latin 'from France'.

This is the French form of Frances q.v. Like the Italian Francesca it dates from the 13th century and probably became established as a Christian name because of the fame of St Francis of Assisi who lived then. See Frances.

Freda

Origin/meaning: Old German 'peaceful friend'.

A short form of Frederica q.v., Alfreda or Winifred q.v. An alternative spelling of Frieda.

Frederica

Origin/meaning: Old German 'peace-rule'.

The feminine form of Frederick q.v. It dates from the 18th century when many masculine names were feminized on the Latin pattern by adding 'a'. Other examples are Augusta and Georgina.

Variations and abbreviations: Federica (It), Fred, Fredi, Freddie, Freddy, Fredericka, Frédérique (Fr), Friederike (Ger), Fritza, Fritzi, Rica, Ricki, Rickie, Ricky, Rikky, Rixi.

Freya

Origin/meaning: Old Norse. The goddess of love and of the night.

Freya was the equivalent in Norse mythology of the Roman goddess Venus. She was the daughter of Niörd, the spirit of water and air and the sister of Frey, the god of fertility. Freya is the name from which the word Friday comes.

Variations and abbreviations: Freia, Freija, Freja, Frigga.

Friday

Origin/meaning: Old Norse 'Freya's day' (Freya was the Norse goddess of love), or old English 'peace-strong' a corruption of Frideswide.

Frideswide (pron. Frids'wid)

Origin/meaning: Old English 'peace-strong'.

One of the few pre-Conquest names which survived the Norman Conquest. St Frideswide, d.735, was daughter of a Mercian king. The name, in several forms which reflected the pronunciation, survived until the general reaction against saints' names after the Protestant Reformation.

Variations and abbreviations: Frediswid, Frévisse (Fr), Friday, Frideswid, Frithswith (Old Eng), Fryswyde.

G

Gabrielle

Origin/meaning: Hebrew 'strong man of God'.

The Italian Gabriella and French/German Gabrielle are fairly recent feminine variations in English-speaking countries.

Variations and abbreviations: Gabey, Gabi, Gabie, Gabriela, Gabriel (Ger), Gabrielle (Fr), Gaby, Gabby, Gavrila (Russ).

Galina

Origin/meaning: Greek 'peace' or 'tranquility'.

A Russian name, which was very fashionable there in the 1960s. Also used in German-speaking countries.

Variations and abbreviations: Gala, Galya.

Gauri

Origin/meaning: Sanskrit 'white'.

In Hindu mythology a name of Shiva's wife, who after being teased by her husband for her dark complexion, meditated until it had turned fair.

Variation: Gowri

Gay

Origin/meaning: French 'merry', 'cheerful'.

This name, taken directly from the adjective, has come into use over the last 100 years.

Variations: Gae, Gaye.

Gaynor

Origin/meaning: Old Welsh 'fair and yielding' or 'white wave'.

This is a form of the Welsh name Guinevere q.v. the name of the wife of King Arthur. It was a form used in Medieval England but then virtually obsolete until the 1950s.

Variations: Gaenor (Wel), Ganor, Gaynore, Guanor (Scot).

Geeta

Origin/meaning: Hindustani 'Holy Book'.

This is the Hindu equivalent of the Bible, being a collection of the sayings of Krishna. The name is found in all regions of India.

Variation: Gita.

Gemma (pron. Jemma)

Origin/meaning: Latin 'jewel'.

Its use in English-speaking countries dates only from this century although it has been a popular Italian name since the Middle Ages.

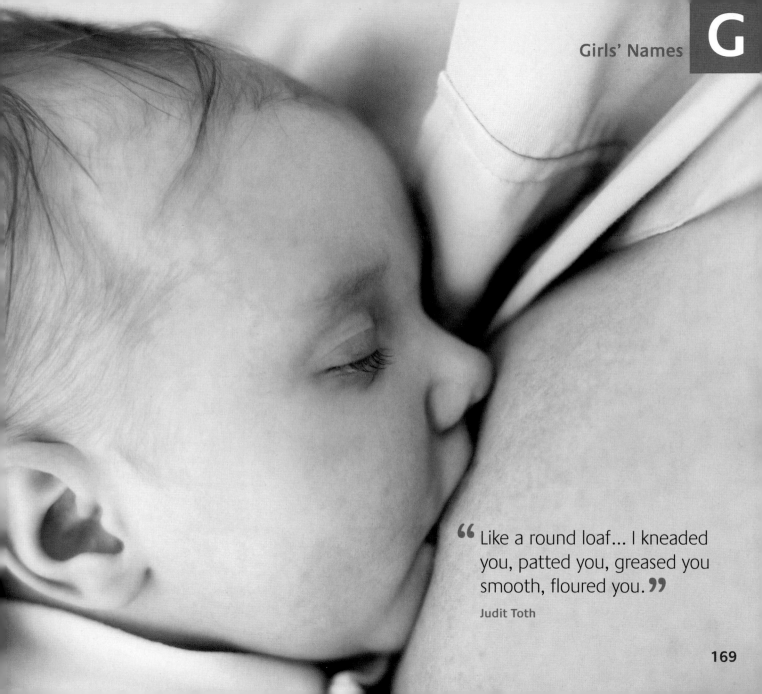

" Like a round loaf... I kneaded you, patted you, greased you smooth, floured you. "

Judit Toth

G

Girls' Names

Genevieve (pron. Jéneveev)
Origin/meaning: uncertain. It includes the Gaulish French word for 'tribe' but the rest is unknown.
This is an old French name, often considered a form or close relative of Guinevere q.v. although in fact their meanings are quite dissimilar. St Geneviève, 420–500, is the patron saint of Paris.
Variations and abbreviations: Geneviève (Fr), Genovefa (Ger), Genoveffa (It), Genoveva, Ginette, Vevo.

Georgette/Georgia
Origin/meaning: Greek 'farmer'.
Feminine forms of George q.v.

Georgiana
Origin/meaning: Greek 'farmer'.
A feminine form of George q.v. By the mid-19th century the slightly simpler form Georgina had superseded it.
Abbreviation: Georgie.

Geraldine
Origin/meaning: Old German 'spear-rule'.
This name originated as an adjective meaning 'of the Fitzgerald family'. Fitzgerald was the family name of the Earls of Kildare. They were descended from the 12th-century Welsh princess Nesta, and Gerald of Windsor. The Earl of Surrey, 1517–1547, fell in love with Lady Elizabeth Fitzgerald and wrote poems to her addressed to 'the Fair Geraldine'. It became really established as a name when Samuel Taylor Coleridge used it in his poem 'Christabel', 1816.
Variations and abbreviations: Geralda, Geralde (Ger), Geraldina, Geraldine (Fr), Gerolda, Gerrie, Gerry, Giralda (It), Jerrie, Jerry.

Gerda
Origin/meaning: Norse mythology. Gerda was the wife of Frey and daughter of the frost giant Gymer.
Frey, the god of Spring, married Gerda, the frozen earth and their children represented the fruitfulness of the earth. Gerda was used by the Danish writer Hans Christian Andersen for his story 'The Snow Queen'.

Germaine
Origin/meaning: Latin 'a German'.
This is the feminine form of German(us) through the French form Germain.
Variation: Germana (It).

Gertrude
Origin/meaning: Old German 'spear-strength'.
This was the name of one of the Valkyries, twelve maidens who accompanied the greatest warriors killed in battle to Valhalla to feast with Odin the chief of the gods. In the Middle Ages the name was popular because of two saints, Gertrude of Nivelles, 626–659, and Gertrude of Helfta, 1256–1302. Many girls were named after them. Shakespeare gave the name to Hamlet's mother in his play 'Hamlet', 1600.

Variations and abbreviations: Gartrude, Gattie, Gatty, Geldrude (It), Gerda, Gertie, Gertraud (Ger), Gertrud (Ger/Scand), Gertruda, Gertrudis (Ger), Gerty, Trudie, Trudy.

Gilda

Origin/meaning: Old English 'golden'.

A medieval name which probably began as a nickname. The name may have been given some extra popularity by the film 'Gilda', 1946, starring Rita Hayworth.

Variations: Golda, Goldie, Goldy.

Gillian

Origin/meaning: from Julius, a Roman family name, possibly meaning 'dowry'.

This name developed in the Middle Ages as a feminine form of Julian. Gillian was one of the most popular medieval names, and has been popular again in Britain from the mid-20th century.

Variations and abbreviations: Gill, Gillet, Gillie, Gilly, Giula (It), Giuletta (It), Giuliana (It), Jillian, Juli, Julia, Juliana, Juliann, Julie (Fr), Julienne, Juliane, Juliet, Julietta, Juliette (Fr), Julita, Julitta.

Gina (pron. Jéena)

Origin/meaning: Latin 'queen'.

This is a short form of Regina, a medieval name. In the 20th century Gina has become accepted as an independent name.

Ginger

Origin/meaning: a pet form of Virginia q.v. or a nickname for people with red hair.

Ginny

Origin/meaning: either Latin from the patrician Roman family Verginius ('Spring') or Latin 'maidenly', 'virginal'.

A short form of Virginia q.v. now commonly used as an independent name.

Gisela

Origin/meaning: Old German 'pledge'.

It has been an independent name for over a thousand years. It is familiar in English-speaking countries because of the ballet 'Giselle', 1841, by the French composer Adolphe Adam.

Variations and abbreviations: Ghislaine, Gila, Gisa, Gisèle (Fr), Giselle, Gisella (It).

Gladys

Origin/meaning: Latin 'lame' from Claudius, the name of two eminent Roman families.

This is one of many Welsh surviving forms of Roman names and in Cornwall, it survived as Gladuse. Gladys has spread outside Wales since the end of the 19th century possibly because it was used by the romantic novelist Ouida in her novel 'Puck', 1870.

Variations and abbreviations: Glad, Gladusa (Cornish), Gladuse (Cornish), Gwladus (Wel), Gwladys (Wel).

Girls' Names

Gloria
Origin/meaning: Latin 'glory'.
Not used as a name until the late 19th century when it seems to have been introduced in the US. Early usage may have been due to the phenomenal popularity of the US film actress Gloria Swanson.

Glynis
Origin/meaning: Welsh Celtic 'valley', 'glen'.
The feminine form of Glyn q.v.
Variations: Glenda, Glenna, Glennis, Glenys, Glynnis, Glynwen.

Godiva
Origin/meaning: Old English 'God's gift'.
Godiva was the wife of Leofric, Earl of Chester, and a generous benefactress of religious institutions. When her husband imposed crippling taxes on the city of Coventry he joked that they would be remitted if she would ride naked through the market place at midday. Godiva took up the challenge and the people of Coventry respected her by remaining indoors while she did so.

Grace
Origin/meaning: Latin 'grace'.
Although used in the Middle Ages this name really established itself in England in the 17th century. Puritans on both sides of the Atlantic used it in the sense of God's favor or bounty. For a long time it was used to 'translate' the native Irish name Gráinne q.v. and was often used where there were Irish connections. Princess Grace of Monaco (Grace Kelly), is an example.
Variations: Engracia (Sp), Gracia (Med Eng), Gracie, Gratia, Gratiana, Grayce, Grazia (It).

Gráinne
Origin/meaning: 'love'.
One of the most popular of the native Irish names brought back into use by the Celtic revival at the beginning of the 20th century. In Irish legend Gráinne was the daughter of Cormac MacArt, one of the five kings of Ulster.
Variations: Grace, Graidhne (Ir), Grainé, Grania.

Greta
Origin/meaning: Persian?/Greek/Latin 'pearl' or French/English 'daisy'.
A German and Scandinavian short form of Margaret q.v. used as an independent name since the 19th century.
Variations: Greda, Greet (Dut), Grete, Gretchen (Ger), Gretel. See also Margaret.

Gudrun
Origin/meaning: Old English 'secret writing'.
Used by D. H. Lawrence in his novel 'Women in Love', 1920. In Scandinavian legend Gudrun was a model of patience.

Guinevere

Origin/meaning: Old Welsh 'fair and yielding' or 'white wave'.

This was the name given to the wife of King Arthur. As a result the name, in varying forms, is found in all the Celtic areas: Wales, Scotland, Ireland, Cornwall, Normandy and Brittany. Guinevere was extremely beautiful (called 'the gray-eyed') and became the much-loved wife of King Arthur but entered into an illicit liaison with Sir Lancelot.

Variations and abbreviations: Gaenor (Wel), Ganor, Gaynor (Med Eng), Gaynore, Genevieve, Ginevre (It), Guener, Guenever, Guenevere, Guenieve, Guenna, Gwenhwyvar (Old Wel), Gwenore (Med Eng), Jenifer (Cor), Jennifer, Vanora (Scot), Wander (Scot).

Gwawl

Origin/meaning: Welsh 'light'.

One of the native names coming back into use in Wales.

Gwen

Origin/meaning: Welsh 'white', 'fair'.

An independent name, the equivalent of the masculine Gwyn, q.v. or a short form of names beginning with that syllable, particularly Gwendolyn q.v.

Variations: Gwenda, Gwenno.

Gwendolyn

Origin/meaning: Welsh 'white (fair) moon/circle/brow'.

Like several other Welsh names, Gwendolyn spread beyond Wales in the 19th century. Sir Walter Scott, in his poem 'The Bridal of Triermain', 1813, probably helped introduce the name to a wider public. In some versions of the Tales of King Arthur, Gwendolyn is the name of Merlin's wife.

Variations and abbreviations: Guendolen, Guendoloena, Guenna, Gwen, Gwenda, Gwendolen (Wel), Gwendolin, Gwennie, Gwynne, Winnie, Wynne.

Gwyneth

Origin/meaning: Welsh 'white/fair maiden'.

This may be the same name as Gyneth, the daughter of King Arthur. Another meaning sometimes given is the area of North Wales known as Gwynedd.

Variations and abbreviations: Gwyn, Gwynaeth, Gwynedd, Gynedd.

H

Hannah

Origin/meaning: Hebrew 'grace', 'graceful'.

The name of the mother of the prophet Samuel.

Variations and abbreviations: Hana, Hanna, Hanni, Hannie, Hanny. See also Ann, Anna, Nancy.

Harriet

Origin/meaning: Old German 'home-ruler'.

An English feminine form of Henry from its Medieval English form Harry. Its main period of popularity was the 18th and 19th centuries.

Variations and abbreviations: Harri, Harrie, Harrietta, Harriette, Harrio, Harriot, Hat, Hattie, Hatty.

Hasina

Origin/meaning: Swahili 'good'.

An East African name.

Variation: Hasanati.

Hayfa

Origin/meaning: Arabic 'slender'.

Hayley

Origin/meaning: Old English 'high clearing'.

A last name used as a first name. It became popular when English actress Hayley Mills was a child star in the late 1950s and early 60s.

Hazel

Origin/meaning: Old German 'hazel-tree'.

One of the many names taken from flowers and trees at the end of the 19th century.

Heather

Origin/meaning: Middle English 'heather'.

It was first used, with many other flower names, at the end of the 19th century.

Hebe (pron. Héebee)

Origin/meaning: Greek 'youth'.

In Greek mythology Hebe was the daughter of Zeus and Hera. She was goddess of youth and Spring and cup-bearer to the gods on Mount Olympus.

> Life is a flame that is always burning itself out, but it catches fire again every time a child is born.

George Bernard Shaw

Girls' Names

Hedda
Origin/meaning: Old German 'struggle'.
A short form of Hedwig q.v. long used in Germany and Scandinavia as an independent name. Ibsen used it for the heroine of his play 'Hedda Gabler', 1890, perhaps because of its meaning.
Variations and abbreviations: see Hedwig.

Hedwig (pron. Hédveeg)
Origin/meaning: Old German 'battle struggle'.
This is the modern German form of a name which has existed for about 1500 years. In English-speaking countries it is best known through its short forms, Hedda and Hedy.
Variations and abbreviations: Avice (Eng), Avis, Edvige (Fr), Edwige (It), Haduwig, Hadwig, Heda, Hedda, Heddy, Hedy, Hedvig (Swed), Hetta, Hetti.

Helen
Origin/meaning: Greek 'light' or 'bright'.
This was the name of an early saint, the Empress Helen(a), 255–330. She was the mother of the Emperor Constantine and is associated with the supposed discovery of the remains of the Holy Cross. In Medieval England and the Celtic areas the name was found as Ellen or Elena, which is closer to the original Greek, Ellayni. However, Helen and Helena were introduced into England during the 16th century. The popularity of the new form may have been in part due to the story of Helen, the wife of the King of Sparta who sparked off the Trojan War by leaving her husband for the Trojan prince Paris.
Variations and abbreviations: Aileen (It), Eileen (Ir), Elaine (Old Fr), Elana, Elane, Elayne, Eleanor, Eleanora, Eleen, Elena (Sp/It), Eleni (Gr), Elenore, Eleonore, Elianora, Elinor, Elinore, Ella, Ellen, Ellene, Ellie, Elly, Ellyn, Elyn, Helena, Helene, Hélène (Fr), Ilene, Lana, Lena, Lenka (Russ), Lenore, Leonora, Nell, Nellie, Nelly.

Helena (pron. Helenuh)
Origin/meaning: Greek 'light' or 'bright'.
The Latinized form of the Greek name Helen q.v. Shakespeare used it in 'A Midsummer Night's Dream' and in 'All's Well That Ends Well'.
Variations and abbreviations: see Helen.

Helga
Origin/meaning: Old Norse 'holy'.
This name was introduced into England by Scandinavian invaders in the 9th century.
Variation: Olga (Russ).

Heloise (pron. Elloweeze)
Origin/meaning: Old German 'flourishing and strong'.
The Norman French version of an Old German name. The usual English form is Eloïse q.v.
Variations and abbreviations: see Eloïse.

Hema
Origin/meaning: Sanskrit 'gold'.
A name found throughout India. The masculine equivalent is Hemchandra.

Henrietta
Origin/meaning: Old German 'home-ruler'.
This is the Latinized form of Henriette, the French feminine form of Henry (Henri). It was introduced into England by the French wife of Charles I. She was really Henriette Marie but became known by the Latin forms of her name Henrietta Maria, 1609–1669.
Variations and abbreviations: Enrichetta (It), Enriquetta (Sp/Port), Etta, Ettie, Etty, Hat, Hattie, Hatty, Heinrike (Ger), Hendrika (Dut), Henka, Hendrickje, Henna, Henrie, Henrieta, Henriette (Fr), Henryetta, Hetti, Hettie, Hetty.

Hermia
Origin/meaning: Greek mythology. Hermes was the messenger of the gods.
This is a feminine form of Hermes. Shakespeare used it for one of the characters in his play 'A Midsummer Night's Dream', 1594. See also Hermione.

Hermione (pron. Hermýohnee)
Origin/meaning: Greek mythology. Hermes was the messenger of the gods.
This, like Hermia q.v. is a feminine form of Hermes. Shakespeare used it for the wife of Leontes in 'The Winter's Tale', 1611 and it has now been made popular by Hermione in the Harry Potter books.

Hero
Origin/meaning: Greek 'chosen one'.
In Greek mythology Hera was the sister/wife of Zeus, the supreme god. She was therefore worshipped as the Queen of the Heavens. Shakespeare used it in 'Much Ado About Nothing', 1598.

Hester
Origin/meaning: uncertain. Probably Persian 'myrtle' or 'star'.
A form of Esther q.v. which was popular in the 17th century.
Variations and abbreviations: Hetty, Hestor.

Hilary
Origin/meaning: Medieval Latin 'cheerful'.
The masculine and feminine forms of this medieval name are the same. The feast day of St Hilary (Hilaire) of Poitiers, 315–367, is January 14th and because of this the first law and university term of the calendar year became known as the Hilary term in the UK.
Variations: Hilaire (Fr), Hilar (Ger), Hilario (Sp/Port), Hilarius (Dut/Ger/Scand), Ilario (It).

Girls' Names

Hilda

Origin/meaning: Old German/Old English 'battle'.

Hild was the chief of the twelve Valkyrie in Norse mythology who rode through battles choosing who was to be slain and taken in glory to Valhalla. Hilda is the Latin version of the original. The name achieved early popularity in England because of St Hilda, 614–680, who founded the famous monastery for both men and women at Whitby in North East England.

Variations: Hild, Hilde, Hildy.

Holly

Origin/meaning: Old English 'holly tree'.

This is one of the flower names which came into fashion at the end of the 19th century. In the film of Truman Capote's novel, 'Breakfast at Tiffany's' Audrey Hepburn played a character called Holly Golightly.

Honey

Origin/meaning: Old English 'nectar'.

During the Middle Ages honey was used instead of sugar to sweeten food and drink and the word became a form of endearment. Honey became popular as a given name after its use by Margaret Mitchell in her 1936 book 'Gone with the Wind'.

Hope

Origin/meaning: Old English 'hope'.

This is one of the three virtues listed by St Paul in his first Epistle to the Corinthians.

Horatia (pron. Horáyshea)

Origin/meaning: Latin, from Horatius, the name of a patrician Roman clan.

The feminine form of Horace/Horatio. This name was given to the daughter (1801–1881) of Lady Hamilton and Admiral Horatio Nelson.

Hyacinth

Origin/meaning: Greek 'hyacinth flower' or 'a red precious stone'.

In Greek mythology, Hyacinth was a beautiful boy loved by the sun god Apollo and Zephyr the West Wind. In English-speaking countries Hyacinth has recently been used as a girl's name as a result of the 19th-century fashion for flower names. The original feminine form was Jacintha q.v.

Variations and abbreviations: see Jacintha.

Hypatia (pron. Hipáyshea)

Origin/meaning: Greek. Uncertain.

In 1853, Charles Kingsley, author of 'The Water Babies', and 'Hereward the Wake', wrote a novel based on the life of Hypatia (375–415) of Alexandria. She was a philosopher and teacher who was respected throughout the known world. As a result of Kingsley's novel, the name has been occasionally used in England.

I

Ianthe (pron. Eeánnthee)
Origin/meaning: Greek 'violet flower'.
A name from Greek mythology; Ianthe was one of the sea nymphs. Byron dedicated his poem 'Childe Harolde', 1817, to Ianthe, a pseudonym for Lady Charlotte Harley. Shelley's daughter, b.1813, was also named Ianthe.
Variation: Iantha. See also Violet and Hyacinth.

Ida
Origin/meaning: Old German 'industrious'.
Possibly derived from an Old German name Idaberga, the name was introduced into England by the Normans. In the 19th century it was revived and its popularity was boosted first by Tennyson's poem 'The Princess', 1847, then by the Gilbert and Sullivan operetta 'Princess Ida', 1884, which was based on it.

Ife (pron. Eefée)
Origin/meaning: Yoruba 'love'.
A popular Nigerian name.
See also Amy, Lerato.

Ignatia (pron. Ignáyshea)
Origin/meaning: uncertain. Possibly Latin 'fiery'.
A feminine form of Ignatius q.v. Usually used by Catholics.

Ila
Origin/meaning: Sanskrit 'world'.

Imogen
Origin/meaning: uncertain. Sometimes given as Old Irish 'girl' or 'daughter' or Greek 'beloved child'.
The regular use of this name in England dates from the present century, although a similar name, Imagina, was used in Europe in the Middle Ages. The source of the modern name is Shakespeare's play 'Cymbeline'. However it appears that Shakespeare had intended Innogen which was definitely an established, though uncommon, name. Imogen therefore appears to be the result of a printer's error, and its meaning is derived from Innogen.
Variations and abbreviations: Imagina, Imogene, Imogine, Immy, Innagon, Innogen.

India
Origin/meaning: Sanskrit 'river' or 'river Indus'.
The name of the country has sometimes been used by people who were born there. It was used for a grand-daughter of Earl Mountbatten, who had been the last Viceroy of India.

I

Girls' Names

Indira
Origin/meaning: Sanskrit 'moon'.
This is based on the same word as the name Indu q.v.

Indu (pron. Indhú)
Origin/meaning: Sanskrit 'moon'.
A common Indian name. Indu was a famous female scholar who lived many thousands of years ago.
See also Chandra, Indira, Selina.

Inez
Origin/meaning: Greek 'pure', 'chaste'.
The Anglicized version of Ines, which is the Spanish equivalent of Agnes, q.v.
Variations: Ines, Inessa, Ynes, Ynez.

Inge
Origin/meaning: Old Norse/Old German Ingvi or Ing, the name of one of the heroes of the Teutonic tribes.
This name is extremely popular in Scandinavia and German-speaking countries. It is frequently used as a double name with others e.g. Inge-Maria. Alternatively it may be a short form of names like Ingrid or Ingeborg.
Variations: Ing, Inga. See also the masculine name Ingmar.

Ingrid
Origin/meaning: Old Norse/Old German 'Ingvi's ride' or 'beloved of Ingvi'.
Another name containing the name of the hero-god Ingvi or Ing. This name has become familiar in English-speaking countries because of the Swedish film actress Ingrid Bergman, 1915–1982.
Abbreviations: Inga, Inge, Inger.

Iona (pron. Eye-ówna)
Origin/meaning: either Greek 'violet coloured stone' or the Scottish Hebridean island.
Although the first meaning is sometimes given, the use of the name in Scotland indicates that the island is its real source. This was the site of St Columba's most important monastery.

Irene (pron. Eiréenee or Éireen)
Origin/meaning: Greek 'peace'.
Eirene is the Greek goddess of peace. Although its use in English-speaking countries is comparatively recent, the name is a very old one. St Irene was burned alive in 304 for refusing to eat food which had been sacrificed to the gods, and for keeping Christian books.
Variations and abbreviations: Eirena, Eirene, Irena, Irina (Slav), Ira, Rena, Rene, Rina.

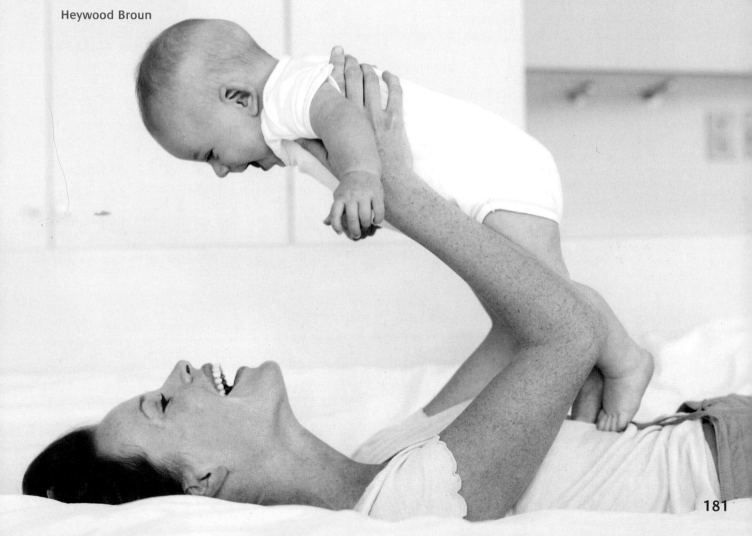
"Except that right side up is best, there is not much to learn about holding a baby. There are one hundred and fifty-two distinctly different ways – and all are right! At least all will do."

Heywood Broun

Girls' Names

Iris
Origin/meaning: Greek 'rainbow'.
In Greek mythology Iris was a goddess who acted as the messenger of the gods. She was personified as a rainbow bridging heaven and earth and the iris flower was given its name because of its rainbow colored varieties.

Irma
Origin/meaning: Old German 'universal'.
This name originated as a pet form of longer names such as Irmtraud and became a first name in English-speaking countries at the end of the 19th century.

Isabel
Origin/meaning: Hebrew 'God is my satisfaction'.
This is an early medieval development of Elizabeth q.v. which began in Spain and Provence. It became Ilsabeth and then Islabeau. Because beau is a masculine adjective it seemed logical to change it, and it became Isabelle in France and in neighboring Spain. The name came to England with Isabella who married King John in 1200. The name was introduced separately into Scotland from France where the usual spelling is Isobel. Isa, Ishbel and Isla are three specifically Scottish short forms.
Variations and abbreviations: Bell, Bella, Belle, Ib, Ibbie, Ibby, Ilsa (Ger), Ilse (Ger), Isa (Scot), Isabeau (Fr), Isabella (It), Isabelle, Isabetta, Ishbel (Scot), Isobel (Scot), Issie, Issy, Izabel, Ysabel.

Isadora
Origin/meaning: uncertain. Possibly Greek 'gift of Isis' (an Egyptian goddess).
The feminine form of an ancient Greek masculine name, Isidore. the name was made famous in the US by the American dancer/choreographer Isadora Duncan, 1878–1927.
Variation: Isidora.

Iseult
Origin/meaning: either Old Welsh 'fair one' or Old German 'ice-rule'.
This is the Celtic form of Isolda q.v.

Ismenia
Origin/meaning: Greek 'learned'.
A medieval name possibly connected with Ismene (pron. Isménee) the daughter of Oedipus and Jocasta.
Variations and abbreviations: Ismay, Ismena, Ismene, Ysmena.

Isolda
Origin/meaning: either Old Welsh 'fair one' or Old German 'ice-rule'.
Isolda is the Latinized form of the German name, while Iseult and its variations which came to England with the Normans, seems to derive from the Celtic/Welsh version which would have been used in the Celtic areas of Normandy and Brittany.

The romantic legend of Tristan and Isolde made it a popular medieval name in the 19th century as did Wagner's opera 'Tristan und Isolde'.

Variations and abbreviations: Essylt, Isaut, Iseut, Iseult, Isold, Isolde (Ger), Isolt, Isota, Yseult, Ysold, Ysolda, Ysolde, Ysolt, Ysonde.

Ivy
Origin/meaning: Old English 'ivy plant'.
One of the flower and plant names which were popular at the end of the 19th century.

J

Jacintha (pron. Jassinta)
Origin/meaning: Greek 'hyacinth flower', 'hyacinth jewel' (red topaz, zircon or garnet).
This is an English version of Hyacinth. It was a Greek name from the mythological character loved by Apollo and killed by Zephyr, the West Wind.
Variations and abbreviations: Cynthia, Cynthie, Giancinta (It), Hyacinth, Hyacintha, Hyacinthe, Hyacinthia, Hyacinthie (Ger), Jacinta (Sp), Jacinthe, Jacynth.

Jacqueline
Origin/meaning: uncertain. Possibly Hebrew 'supplanter'.
This is a feminine form of James from the French Jacques. It was used in the Middle Ages but has been most popular in the 20th century.
Variations and abbreviations: Jacki, Jackie, Jacky, Jaclyn, Jacquelyn, Jacqui. See also Jacquetta.

Jacquetta
Origin/meaning: uncertain. Possibly Hebrew 'supplanter'.
A French feminine form of James from the French masculine form Jacques. It was known in the Middle Ages and Shakespeare used it in 'Love's Labour's Lost', 1594.
Variations: Jacquenetta, Jacquenette, Jacquette, Jaquetta.

Jade
Origin/meaning: Old French/Spanish 'jade', a semi-precious stone.
Used as a name since the late 19th century when gem names became fashionable.
Variation: Ijada (Sp).

Girls' Names

Jameela
Origin/meaning: Arabic 'beautiful'.
A popular Muslim name.
Variation: Jamila. See also Belle.

Jane
Origin/meaning: Hebrew 'Jehovah has favored'.
This feminine form of John came into fashion in England in the 16th century. It usurped Joan, the original native form.
Variations: Jana, Janey, Janie, Jayne. See also Joan.

Janet
Origin/meaning: 'Little Jane' a diminutive of Jane. Hebrew 'Jehovah has favored'.
This has long been an independent name rather than a mere pet form of Jane. It was originally associated with Scotland.
Variations and abbreviations: Jennet (Med Eng), Jonet, Netta, Nettie. See also Joan.

Janice
Origin/meaning: Hebrew 'Jehovah has favored'.
A US form of Joan, probably from Jan, the short form of another variation, Jane. It has now spread to other English-speaking countries.
Variation: Janis. See also Joan.

Jasmine
Origin/meaning: Arabic/Persian 'jasmine flower'.
This is the English version of the Arabic Yasmin. Like other flower names it came into use at the end of the 19th century.
Variations and abbreviations: Gelsomina (It), Jasmin (Ger), Jasmina, Jessamine (Fr), Jessamy, Jessamyn, Jess, Jessie, Jessy, Yasmin (Arab).

Jayanti
Origin/meaning: Sanskrit 'victorious'.
The feminine form of Jayant, and found in Hindu texts as an epithet of Durga, Shiva's wife, and as the name of Indra's daughter. Jayanti is often used to denote the anniversary of a birth or death.

Jayashree
Origin/meaning: Sanskrit 'victory'.
A popular Indian name.

Jean
Origin/meaning: Hebrew 'Jehovah has favored'.
This is a Scottish form of the English name Joan. Jean comes via the Old French form Jehane which was used in Scotland because of the close ties between Scotland and France.
Variations: Jeanie, Jeanne (Fr), Jeannette.

Jemima

Origin/meaning: Hebrew 'dove'.
This is a 17th-century Biblical name. Jemima was one of Job's three daughters.
Variations and abbreviations: Jamima, Jem, Jemie, Jemmie, Jemmy, Mimie.

Jennie/Jenny

Origin/meaning: since the 1920s this has been the most common as a short form of the newly fashionable name Jennifer. Prior to that it was considered a familiar form of Jane or Jean. Jennie (Jeannette) Jerome, was an American heiress who married Lord Randolph Churchill, 1874, and was the mother of Sir Winston Churchill.

Jennifer

Origin/meaning: Old Welsh 'fair and yielding' or 'white wave'.
This is the Cornish form of the Old Welsh name Gwenhywvar (Guinevere). Variations of Guinevere were found in all the Celtic areas, including Cornwall, for the Tales of King Arthur formed an integral part of their folklore. It appeared in the rest of England in the 1920s and is very popular in the US.
Variations and abbreviations: Jen, Jenifer, Jenni, Jenny. See also Guinevere.

Jessica

Origin/meaning: Hebrew 'God beholds'.
Used by Shakespeare as the name of Shylock's daughter in 'The Merchant of Venice'. It is probably a version of the Biblical Iscah. Rare, even among Jewish people, until the mid-20th century, now very popular.
Variations and abbreviations: Gessica (It), Jesca, Jess, Jessalin, Jessie, Jessy.

Jessie

Origin/meaning: Hebrew 'Jehovah has favored'.
A Scottish short form of Janet, itself a feminine form of John. Now found as an independent name. Sometimes used as a short form of Jessica or Jasmine q.v.
Variations and abbreviations: Jess, Jessy.

Jill

Origin/meaning: from Julius, a Roman family name, possibly meaning 'dowry'.
This short form of Gillian/Jillian/Juliana has been used since the Middle Ages. It is currently popular as an independent name.

Joan

Origin/meaning: Hebrew 'Jehovah has favored'.
The most usual Medieval English feminine form of John q.v. It was often spelt Johan.
Variations and abbreviations: Gianna (It), Giannina (It), Giovanna (It), Hanna (Ger), Jan, Jana (US), Janella, Janelle, Janet, Janetta, Janette, Janey, Jania, Janice, Janie, Janine, Janis, Janith, Janka, Janna (Ger), Jannelle, Jany, Janyte, Jayne, Jean (Scot), Jeanette (Fr),

Girls' Names

Jeanie, Jeanne (Fr), Jeannette (Fr), Jeannine (Fr), Jennet, Jenni, Jennie, Jenny, Jenyth, Jess, Jessie, Jessy, Jinny, Jo-Ann, Joan, Joana, Joanna, Joanne (Fr), Johanna (Ger), Joni, Jonie, Juana (Sp/Port), Juanita (Sp/Port), Netta, Nettie, Shena (Scot), Sheena (Scot), Sian (Wel), Siné (Scot), Sinead (Ir).

Joanna

Origin/meaning: Hebrew 'Jehovah has favored'.
This is the Latinized version of the medieval feminine form of John, Joan. It was sometimes used in the Middle Ages. In the 18th century Joanna was used as an independent name when Latinized endings for feminine names were fashionable. In the mid-20th century Joanne, the French version, became more popular.
Variations and abbreviations: Jo, Joana, Jo-Ann, Joanne (Fr), Johanna (Ger).

Jocasta

Origin/meaning: Greek 'shining moon'.
In Greek legend Jocasta is the mother of Oedipus who unwittingly kills his father and marries his mother.

Jocelyn

Origin/meaning: Old German 'man of the Goths'.
This pre-Conquest name was introduced into England by the Normans and until the 20th century was used exclusively as a male name. Recently, probably because of its similarity to two other feminine names, Joyce and Lynn, it has been used for girls rather than boys.
Variations and abbreviations: Joceline, Josceline, Joscelyn, Joss, Josselyn, Joycelin.

Jodi/Jody

Origin/meaning: Hebrew 'Jewish woman', 'from Judah'.
A modern diminutive of Judith q.v., currently a vogue name in North America, where it originated.
Variations: Jodie. See also Judith.

Joelle

Origin/meaning: Hebrew 'Jehovah is god'.
A US feminine form of Joel q.v. created by adding a typical French feminine ending.
Variations: Joella, Joellen.

Jonquil

Origin/meaning: the name of a flower similar to the narcissus.
This is one of the more unusual flower names which became popular at the end of the 19th century.

Jordan

Origin/meaning: Hebrew 'flowing down'.
Jordan has been used as a masculine and feminine name since the Crusaders brought back the name of this river from the Holy Land in the Middle Ages.

Birth is the sudden opening of a window, through which you look out upon a stupendous prospect. For what has happened? A miracle. You have exchanged nothing for the possibility of everything.

William MacNeile Dixon

Girls' Names

Josephine

Origin/meaning: Hebrew 'May Jehovah increase'.
This is a French feminine diminutive form of Joseph q.v. The name came into use at the beginning of the 19th century because of Napoleon Bonaparte's wife (1763–1814), known throughout Europe as the Empress Josephine.
Variations and abbreviations: Fifi, Fina, Giuseppa (It), Giuseppina (It), Jo, Jo-Jo, Jolene (US), Josée (Fr), Josefa (Ger), Josefina (Sp/Port), Josefine, Josepha, Joséphine (Fr), Josette, Josie, Josy, Pepita (Sp), Peppina (It).

Josie

Origin/meaning: Hebrew 'May Jehovah increase'.
A short form of Josephine used mainly in the US.
Variations: Josy. See also Josephine.

Joy

Origin/meaning: Latin 'rejoicing', French 'joy'.
A medieval Christian name.

Joyce

Origin/meaning: French Celtic 'champion'.
The English form of Judoc(us), or Josse, the name of a 7th-century Breton saint, whose relics were brought to the newly built Minster of Winchester in the 10th century. Like many medieval names the same form was used for men and women. Later it become an almost exclusively feminine name.
Variations: Joice, Joisse (Med Fr), Josse (Med Eng), Joycelin.

Judith

Origin/meaning: Hebrew 'Jewish woman', 'from Judah'.
Judith was the heroine of the Apocryphal Book of Judith. She saved the town of Bethulia by seducing Nebuchadnezzar's general Holofernes and then cutting off his head while he slept. Although there are several medieval examples including a niece of William the Conqueror, it did not become popular in Britain until the 17th century.
Variations and abbreviations: Giuditta (It), Jodi, Jodie, Jody, Judi, Judie, Judintha, Juditha (Ger), Judy, Judye, Jutta.

Julia

Origin/meaning: from Julius, a Roman family name, possibly meaning 'dowry'.
This is the direct equivalent of the masculine Julius. It may have been Shakespeare who introduced the name into England when he used it for the Italian Giulia in his play 'Two Gentlemen of Verona', 1598. The name is sometimes used for girls born in July, the month named after Julius Caesar.
Variations and abbreviations: Giulia (It), Jule, Jules, Julie (Fr).

Juliana

Origin/meaning: from Julius, a Roman family name possibly meaning 'dowry'.
The Latin feminine version of Julian q.v.
Variations and abbreviations: Giuliana (It), Juliane, Julianne, Julienne, Julie.

Julie

Origin/meaning: from the Roman family name Julius, possibly meaning 'dowry'.
The French form of Julia q.v., which became very popular in English-speaking countries in the 20th century.
Variations and abbreviations: see Julia.

Juliet

Origin/meaning: 'little Julia'. From the Roman family name Julius, possibly meaning 'dowry'.
Shakespeare based his play 'Romeo and Juliet' on a poem by Arthur Brooke called 'The Tragical History of Romeus and Juliet',
1562. Brooke had presumably 'translated' the Italian name Giuletta.
Variations and abbreviations: Jule, Juliette (Fr). See also Gillian.

Jumoke (pron. J'mókhi)

Origin/meaning: Yoruba 'everyone loves the child'.
A Nigerian name that can be used for both boys and girls.

June

Origin/meaning: the sixth month of the year.
The month may have taken its name from Juno, the Chief of the goddesses and the patron of all female concerns from birth to death. The name June has come into use in the 20th century with one or two examples in the 19th century.

Juno

Origin/meaning: Old Irish, uncertain, possibly 'lamb'.
A variation of Oonagh q.v. best known for Sean O'Casey's play 'Juno and the Paycock', 1924.

Justine

Origin/meaning: Latin 'just'.
The French feminine version of Justin q.v.
Variations: Giustina (It), Justina (Sp).

Kailas (pron. Kyelahs)

Origin/meaning: Sanskrit. The name of a holy mountain in the Himalayas.
Hindus believe that the God Shiva and Parvati q.v. his wife live on Mount Kailas.

Kamala

Origin/meaning: Sanskrit 'pale red'.
The feminine form of Kamal and found often in Hindu classical texts, including as a name of the goddess Lakshami, wife of Vishnu.

Kamaria (pron. Kamaréea)

Origin/meaning: Swahili 'moon-like'.
A popular name in East Africa.

Karen

Origin/meaning: uncertain. Possibly Greek 'pure'.
A Scandinavian form of Katharine q.v. It was introduced into the US by Scandinavian immigrants and has subsequently spread to other English-speaking countries.
Variations: Caren, Carin, Karim. See also Katharine.

Kashmira

Origin/meaning: Kashmin 'from Kashmir'.
A name given because Kashmir is considered a holy area.

Kate

Origin/meaning: uncertain. Possibly Greek 'pure'.
This is a short form of Katharine q.v. Shakespeare's Katherina Minola, the 'Shrew' of his play 'The Taming of the Shrew', 1594, is referred to as Kate. The name was again popular in the 19th century when Susan Coolidge (1835–1905) the US children's writer, wrote her Katy books.
Variations: Katie, Katy. See also Katharine.

Katharine/Katherine

Origin/meaning: uncertain. Possibly Greek 'pure'.
Tradition has it that Katherine of Alexandria was one of the virgin martyrs who died in Alexandria early in the 4th century after protesting about the worship of idols. Attempts were made to torture her into submission including the spiked 'Catherine wheel'

which miraculously disintegrated beneath her. Eventually Katherine was beheaded. Her body was carried by angels to Mount Sinai, where a church was built in her honor.

Variations and abbreviations: Caitlin (Ir), Caitrin, Caren, Carin, Caryn, Cass, Cassie, Cassy, Catalina (Sp), Catarina, Cate, Catelin (Med Eng), Caterina (It), Catharina, Catharine, Cathee, Catherina, Catherine (Fr), Cathie, Cathleen (Ir), Cathlene, Cathrine, Cathryn, Cathy, Catia (It), Catie, Catlin (Med Eng), Catriona (Scot), Caty, Ekaterina (Ger/Russ), Karen (Scand), Karin, Kass, Kassia, Kassie, Kata, Katalin, Kate, Katerina, Katerine, Katey, Katha, Katharina (Ger), Kathi, Kathie, Kathleen (Ir), Kathryn, Kathy, Katia (Ger), Katie, Katina, Katinka (Russ), Katja (Russ), Katrina (Gk), Katrinka, Katya, Kay, Kaye, Kit, Kittie, Kitty, Treena, Trina.

Kathleen

Origin/meaning: uncertain. Possibly Greek 'pure'.
The Irish diminutive form of Katharine q.v.
Variations and abbreviations: Cath, Cathee, Cathleen, Cathie, Catty, Kay, Kath, Kathie, Kathy. See also Katharine.

Kay

Origin/meaning: uncertain. Possibly Greek 'pure'.
A short form of Katharine q.v.

Keira

Origin/meaning: Old Irish 'dark haired'.
A variation of Ciara that has become known because of the British actress Keira Knightley.

Kelly

Origin/meaning: Gaelic 'descendant of War'.
Celtic surname most commonly found in Ireland, now popular as a girl's first name. It is very popular in the US, especially among Americans with Irish descent.
Variation: Kellie.

Kerrie

Origin/meaning: 'from Kerry', an Irish place-name, meaning the place of dark-haired people.
Variations: Keriann, Kerianne, Kerry, Kerryn. See also Kieran.

Kezia

Origin/meaning: Hebrew 'cassia' (a type of cinnamon).
Kezia was one of the three beautiful daughters of Job. The name was used by the Puritans.
Variation: Keziah.

Khadija

Origin/meaning: Arabic 'born prematurely'.
Khadija was the wife of Mohammed.
Variation: Kedeja.

Girls' Names

Kibibi
Origin/meaning: Swahili 'little lady'.
An East African name.
See also Martha.

Kim
Origin/meaning: Old English 'cyne' – 'royal'. From the surname Kimball 'royal hill' or Kimberley 'royal meadow'.
This name became popular for boys after the publication in 1901 of Rudyard Kipling's book 'Kim'. It has now become equally popular for girls.

Kimberley
Origin/meaning: Old English 'from the royal meadow'.
This is an English last name which has become popular as a girl's name in the US and Australia.
Variations and abbreviations: Kim, Kimmie.

Kirsten
Origin/meaning: Latin 'Christian'.
The Scandinavian form of the English names Christine, Christina and Christiana.
Variations and abbreviations: Kerstin, Kerstina, Kirsteen (Scot), Kirsty, Kris, Krissy, Kirstin, Kristin, Kristina, Kristine. See also Christiana, Christine.

Kirsty
Origin/meaning: Latin 'Christian'.
This is a Scottish pet form of Christine/Christiana. It comes from the Scandinavian form Kirsten.
Variations: Kirstie. See also Kirsten and Christine.

Kitty
Origin/meaning: uncertain. Possibly Greek 'pure'.
A pet form of Katharine q.v.

Kumari
Origin/meaning: Sanskrit 'maiden, daughter'.
A feminine form of Kumar that is found throughout Hindu texts.

Kusum (pron. Kuhsoom)
Origin/meaning: Sanskrit 'flower'.
Popular throughout India.
Variation: Kusum kumari.

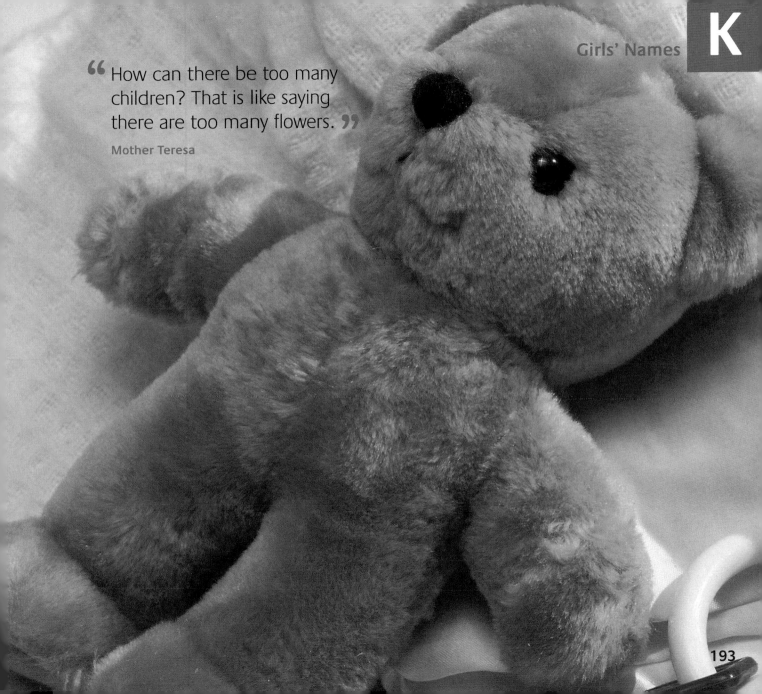

"How can there be too many children? That is like saying there are too many flowers. "

Mother Teresa

Girls' Names

Kyle
Origin/meaning: Gaelic 'narrow strait or sound'.
This is a place-name from Scotland which has become a last name. In the latter half of the 20th century it was used as a feminine first name, particularly in the US. The familiar form Kylie is a native word in Western Australia for a boomerang.
Variations: Kylie, Kyly.

L

Laetitia (pron. Letisha)
Origin/meaning: Latin 'joy', 'delight'.
Laetitia was found occasionally in the Middle Ages but did not really establish itself until the 18th century.
Variations and abbreviations: Lätitia (Ger), Lece (Fr), Lecia, Leda, Letice, Leticia, Letitia, Letizia (It), Lettice (Eng), Letty.

Lakshmi (pron. L'kshmee)
Origin/meaning: Hindu. The name of the goddess of wealth and prosperity, the wife of Vishnu.

Lalita
Origin/meaning: Sanskrit 'playful'.
A name found in Hindu texts, in particular as the name of the female cowherd who became a playmate of the adolescent Krishna.
Variation: Lalit.

Lana
Origin/meaning: a short form of either Helen (Greek 'light' or 'bright') or Alanna (Celtic 'beautiful').

Lara
Origin/meaning: uncertain. Possibly Greek 'cheerful'.
A Russian short form of Larissa q.v. Byron used it for his poem 'Lara', 1814. It may well have been popularized more recently by Pasternak's best-selling book 'Doctor Zhivago', which was also a successful film, for Lara is the heroine of Pasternak's novel.
Variations and abbreviations: See Larissa.

Larissa
Origin/meaning: uncertain. Possibly Greek 'cheerful' or Pre-Hellenic 'castle'.
Larissa, with the short form Lara, has been one of the most popular names in the Soviet Union since the 1960s.
Variations and abbreviations: Lara, Larisa.

Lata (pron. L'ta)
Origin/meaning: Sanskrit 'climbing plant', 'bower'.

Laura
Origin/meaning: Latin 'bay tree' or 'from Laurentium' (city of laurels).
A feminine form of Laurence q.v. which probably evolved as a short form of the cumbersome original Laurencia.
Variations and abbreviations: Laure (Fr), Laureen, Laurel, Lauren, Laurence (Fr), Laurencia, Laurenzia, Lauretta (It), Laurette, Laurie, Laurine, Lora (It), Loreen, Loren, Lorene, Lorenza (It), Loretta, Lorette (Fr), Lori, Lorrie.

Laurel
Origin/meaning: Latin 'laurel' or 'bay tree'.
Used in the 19th century when flower names were in vogue. Laurel symbolizes victory and peace. The laurel/bay was also associated with poetry.
Variations and abbreviations: See Laura.

Lauren
Origin/meaning: Latin 'bay tree' or 'from Laurentium' (city of laurels).
Like Laura this is a short form of Laurencia, the feminine form of Laurence q.v.
Variations and abbreviations: See Laura.

Lavinia
Origin/meaning: uncertain. Possibly 'from Lavinium' (a town near Rome). Sometimes given as 'purified'.
Lavinia is a name from Roman literature. In Virgil's poem the 'Aeneid' Aeneas, a Trojan hero, escapes after the fall of Troy and after many years of wandering reaches Italy. He allies with Latinus whose daughter Lavinia he marries. Their son, Romulus, eventually becomes the founder of Rome. Shakespeare gave the name to the daughter of Titus Andronicus in his play of the same name, 1589, and that is probably the source of modern usage.
Abbreviation: Leni.

Layla
Origin/meaning: Arabic 'intoxicating'.
In Arab literature, the story by 7th-century poet Qays Ibn al-Mulawwah about his love for his cousin Layla is as well known as Romeo and Juliet and their names are similarly associated with love and devotion.

Leah
Origin/meaning: Hebrew 'heifer'. Sometimes given as 'weary'.
Leah was the first wife of Jacob, one of the patriarchs of the Old Testament.

L

Girls' Names

Lee
Origin/meaning: Old English 'meadow'.
An English last name adopted in the 19th century as a first name. Originally a masculine name it is now used equally for girls.
Variations: Lea, Leigh.

Leela
Origin/meaning: Sanskrit 'play'.
Found in Hindu texts, it is associated with amorous sport or feigning love.

Leila (pron. Layla)
Origin/meaning: Persian 'night' or 'dark-haired as night'.
A popular Muslim name. It is found in the Persian legend of Leila and Majnoun. Byron used the name for a beautiful young concubine in his poem 'The Giaour', which introduced Leila as a name to English-speaking countries.
Variations: Layla, Leilah, Lela, Lelah, Lila.

Lena
Origin/meaning: Greek 'light' or 'bright' or Hebrew 'Woman of Magdala'.
A short form of Helena, now an independent name. When pronounced Layna it is a short form of Magdalena.
Variation: Leni.

Léonie
Origin/meaning: Greek 'lion'.
A French feminine form of the popular French name Leon q.v.
Variations and abbreviations: Leo, Leona, Leonia (It), Leonzia (It).

Leonora
Origin/meaning: Greek 'bright', 'light'.
An Italian form of Eleanor/a q.v. similar to the German name Lenore.
Variations and abbreviations: Leonore (Ger), Leonor, Lora.

Lerato
Origin/meaning: Tswana 'love'.
A name from Botswana in South Africa.
See also Amy, Ife.

Lesley
Origin/meaning: Scots Gaelic 'garden by the pool'.
This spelling of the Scottish last name is generally the one used for girls. The first use of Lesley as a first name seems to be for Lesley Baillie, the 'Bonnie Lesley' of the poem by Robert Burns, 1759–1796.
Variations and abbreviations: Les, Lesli, Leslie, Lesly, Lezley, Lezlie.

Lettice

Origin/meaning: Latin 'joy', 'delight'.

The English form of Laetitia q.v. It was extremely popular throughout the Middle Ages.

Variations and abbreviations: see Laetitia.

Libby

Origin/meaning: Hebrew 'God is my satisfaction'.

A short form of Elizabeth q.v. sometimes given as an independent name.

Variations and abbreviations: Lib, Libbie. See also Elizabeth.

Liesl

Origin/meaning: Hebrew 'God is my satisfaction'.

A variation of Elizabeth that was the name of the eldest child in the 1965 Oscar-winning musical 'The Sound of Music'.

Lilith

Origin/meaning: Hebrew 'belonging to the night' or Assyrian 'goddess of storms'.

In non-Biblical Hebrew mythology, Lilith was a wife of Adam before he gave his rib to create Eve.

Lillian

Origin/meaning: Hebrew 'God is my satisfaction'.

This is one of dozens of variations of the name Elizabeth.

Variations and abbreviations: Lili, Lilian, Liliane, Lilias (Scot), Lilla, Lilli (Ger), Lillias (Scot), Lillie, Lilyan.

Lily

Origin/meaning: Greek 'lily' or pet form of Elizabeth (Hebrew 'God is my satisfaction').

In use since the late 19th century fashion for flower names.

Variations and abbreviations: Lil, Lilli, Lillie, Lilly. See also Susannah and Elizabeth.

Linda

Origin/meaning: Old German 'serpent'.

Linda is a short form of the many pre-Conquest names which contained the word. The best known nowadays are Belinda and Rosalind. Serpent may seem a strange meaning but in fact it was very flattering. In German mythology the serpent was regarded as a magical creature. Linda is also the Spanish word for pretty.

Variations: Lindi, Lindy, Lynda.

Lindsay

Origin/meaning: Old English. Uncertain, possibly 'Lincoln's island'.

A Scottish aristocratic last name adopted as a male and female first name.

Variations and abbreviations: Lin, Lindsey (Eng), Linsay, Linsey, Lyn, Lynsey.

Girls' Names

Lisa/Liza

Origin/meaning: Hebrew 'God is my satisfaction'.
Short forms of Elizabeth.
Variations: Elisa, Elise, Eliza, Elizabeth, Lissa.

Lois (pron. Lóys or Lówis)

Origin/meaning: Greek, meaning uncertain.
A Biblical name taken by 17th-century Puritans. Lois Lane is the girlfriend of the comic-strip character Superman.

Lola

Origin/meaning: a Spanish diminutive of Dolores (Spanish 'sorrows') or Carlota (the Spanish form of Charlotte 'man').
Variation: Lolita.

Lorna

Origin/meaning: this name was invented by the novelist R. D. Blackmore for his classic novel 'Lorna Doone', 1869. The name was apparently adapted from the title of the Marquess of Lorne.
See also Fiona, Miranda, Ophelia, Pamela, Perdita, Vanessa and Wendy.

Lorraine

Origin/meaning: French 'from Lorraine' (an area of France).
This has only come into use since the middle of the 20th century. Even in France it is an unusual name.
Variations and abbreviations: Larain, Lorain, Loraine, Lorri, Lorrayne.

Lottie

Origin/meaning: Old German 'man', by association 'womanly'.
A common familiar form (like Tottie) of Charlotte, a feminine form of Charles q.v.
Variations: Lotte, Lotty. See also Charlotte.

Louisa/Louise

Origin/meaning: Old German 'glorious battle'.
These are the Latin and French feminine forms of the French name Louis q.v.
Variations and abbreviations: Lodovica (It), Loise, Lou, Louie, Louise (Fr), Louisette, Lu, Ludowika (Ger), Luigia (It), Luisa (It/Sp), Luise (Ger), Lulu.

Lourdes

Origin/meaning: from the place where St Bernadette of Lourdes, 1844–1879, the miller's daughter claimed to see visions of the Virgin Mary and where today healing miracles take place. It has become familiar as a given name after the singer Madonna named her daughter Lourdes.

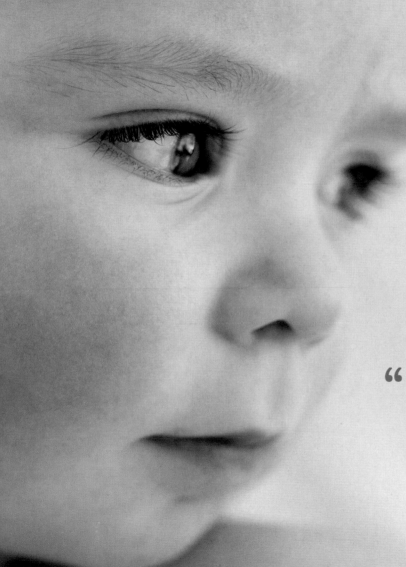

66 Babies are bits of star-dust blown from the Hand of God. Lucky the woman who knows the pangs of birth for she has held a star. 99

Larry Barretto, The Indiscreet Years

Girls' Names

Loveday
Origin/meaning: Medieval English 'born on loveday'.
A loveday was an annual day set aside for settling disputes. In the 17th century it also came to mean a day when the young people of a town or village could look for a partner.

Lubna
Origin/meaning: Arabic 'storax tree'.
Taken from the tree with sweet sap that is used to make incense and perfume. Lubna is the heroine of a famous Arab love story.

Lucasta (pron. Lookásta)
Origin/meaning: Latin 'light'.
A poetic form of Lucia/Lucy q.v. used in the 17th century.
See also Lucy and Althea.

Lucia
Origin/meaning: Latin 'light'.
The original Latin feminine form of Lucius q.v. from which the English Lucy and French Lucille are derived.
Variations and abbreviations: see Lucy.

Lucinda
Origin/meaning: Latin 'light'.
This is a 17th-century form of Lucy.
Variations: Lucinde. See also Lucy.

Lucretia
Origin/meaning: Latin, belonging to the Roman family Lucretius.
This is a classical name revived in Italy during the Renaissance period and used in England mainly from the 16th–18th centuries.
Variations: Lucrèce (Fr), Lucrecia (Sp), Lucresse, Lucrezia (It).

Lucy
Origin/meaning: Latin 'light'.
Lucy is the English form of Lucia, a Roman name. St Lucia, d.304 was a virgin martyr who met her death at Syracuse in Sicily during one of the persecutions by the Emperor Diocletian. She is a saint invoked against eye disease.
Variations and abbreviations: Luc, Lucasta (17th century), Luce (It), Lucetta, Lucette, Luci, Lucia (Ger/It/Lat), Luciana (It), Lucienne (Fr), Lucilia, Lucilla (It), Lucille (Fr), Lucina (It), Lucinda (17th century), Lucinde, Lucine, Lucky (US), Luz, Luzi, Luzia (Ger).

Lulu
Origin/meaning: Old German 'glorious battle', Arabic 'pearl'.
A pet form of Louisa/Louise q.v. or a Muslim name quite unconnected with the European name.

Lydia
Origin/meaning: Greek 'from Lydia' (an ancient kingdom of Asia Minor renowned for its wealthy King, Croesus). This pre-Christian name occurs in the Acts of the Apostles. Lydia was sometimes said to be a daughter of Joseph of Nazareth. Jane Austen used the name for one of Mrs Bennet's daughters in 'Pride and Prejudice', 1813.

Lynn/Lynne
Origin/meaning: Old English 'pool' or a short form of the Welsh Eluned q.v. Possibly 'idol'.
The short form, now used independently, of Eluned or its French variation Lynette, which came into general use in the 19th century.
Variations: Lyn , Lynette.

Lynnet
Origin/meaning: uncertain. Possibly connected with the Old Welsh word meaning 'idol'.
This is a variation of the well-established Welsh name Eluned q.v. from the short form, which is Lyn. It was Tennyson who first used the spelling Lynnet.
Variations and abbreviations: Eiluned, Elined, Eluned, Linet, Linette, Linnet, Luned, Lyn, Lynelle, Lynette, Lynne, Lynnet, Lynnette.

Lysia
Origin/meaning: uncertain.
This is the traditional name given to the twin of St Thomas the Apostle.
See Thomas.

M

Madeleine
Origin/meaning: Hebrew 'woman from Magdala'.
This name comes from a corruption of Magdalene. The old pronunciation was 'maudlin' which, because Mary Magdalene was patron saint of penitents, came to mean tearful. Both spelling and pronunciation were supplanted by the French form of Madeleine.
Variations and abbreviations: Mad, Maddelena (It), Maddie, Maddy, Madeline (Eng), Madelon (Fr), Madeline (US, Madlen, Madlon, Mado, Magda, Magdalena (Ger/Lat/Scand), Magdalene (Eng), Magdelone (Dan), Malena, Malina, Lena, Lene.

Madhur
Origin/meaning: Sanskrit 'sweet'.
A word usually used to describe sounds and tastes that has recently become a given name.

M

Girls' Names

Madhuri (pron. Madtoorée)

Origin/meaning: Sanskrit 'sweet'.

This name comes from madhu, the Sanskrit word for honey or spring.

See also Dulcie, Mandisa and the masculine name Madhukar.

Madonna

Origin/meaning: Latin 'my lady'.

An honorific title for the Virgin Mary that started being used as a given name in America amongst those of Italian descent. Since the 1980s it has become well known for being the name of the singer Madonna Ciccone.

Maeve

Origin/meaning: Old Irish, meaning uncertain.

Maedbh was Queen of Connaught in the 3rd century who fought a great battle over a brown bull, the subject of an epic poem.

Maia (pron. Mýuh)

Origin/meaning: Latin 'exalted'.

The name of a Roman goddess, the mother of Mercury. She may be based on a more ancient Indian deity, associated with visions. This Italian name is sometimes considered the equivalent of the English name May, as that month is thought by some to have been named after the goddess.

Variations: Maija (Fin), Maja (Ger/Scand).

Maida

Origin/meaning: Old English 'maiden, virgin'.

Variation: Mayda

Mandisa (pron. Mandéeza)

Origin/meaning: Xhosa 'sweet'.

A name from the South of Africa.

Mara

Origin/meaning: Hebrew 'bitter'.

A form of the Hebrew name usually translated as Mary or Miriam.

Variations: Marah

Marcella

Origin/meaning: Latin 'little Marcus' from the name of Mars the Roman god of war.

Marcella, the feminine form, has been used occasionally in English-speaking countries.

Variations: Marcella (Sp), Marcelia, Marceline, Marcelle (Fr), Marcellina (It), Marcelline. See also Marcia and Martina.

Marcia (pron. Márssia or Marsha)

Origin/meaning: 'of Mars' (the Roman god of war) i.e. 'warlike'.

This name comes from the Roman family name Marcius. Marcia was the oldest daughter in the classic US sitcom, 'The Brady Bunch' (1969–1974).

Variations and abbreviations: Marcelia, Marcie (Fr), Marcy, Marquita, Marsha (US).

Margaret

Origin/meaning: Persian?/Greek/Latin 'pearl' or Medieval French/English 'daisy'.

The first meaning is probably the correct meaning of this name, although Margaret is an old word for daisy in English and Marguerite, the French form, is also the word for an ox-eye daisy. St Margaret of Scotland, 1045–1093, ensured that the name endured. When Queen Elizabeth the Queen Mother gave birth to her second daughter at Glamis Castle in Scotland she was named Margaret, for she was the first child in direct succession to the throne to be born in Scotland for 300 years.

Variations and abbreviations: Daisy, Greta, Gretel, Gritty, Madge, Mag, Maggie, Maggs, Maggy, Maisie, Mamie, Margareta (Swed/Ger), Margarete (Ger/Dan), Margaretha (Dut/Ger), Margarette, Margarita (Sp), Margaux, Marge, Marged (Wel), Margery, Marget, Marghanita, Margherita (It), Margie, Margit (Swed), Margita (Swed), Margo, Margot, Margred (Wel), Margrethe (Dan), Margriet, Marguerita, Marguerite (Fr), Margy, Marina, Marjie, Marjorie, Marjory, May, Meg, Megan (Wel), Meggie, Meggy, Meghan, Megs, Meta, Mog, Peg, Pegeen, Peggi, Peggie, Peggoty, Rita.

Margery

Origin/meaning: Persian?/Greek/Latin 'pearl' or French/English 'daisy'.

An alternative English spelling of Marjorie q.v. which is a form of Margaret q.v.

Variations and abbreviations: see Margaret.

Marguerite

Origin/meaning: Persian?/Greek/Latin 'pearl' or French/English 'daisy'.

This is the French form of Margaret q.v.

Variations and abbreviations: see Margaret.

Maria

Origin/meaning: uncertain. Possibly Hebrew 'bitter' or 'wished for child'.

The Latin form of Mary used to translate the original Hebrew Mrym. All other forms of the name stem from it.

Variations and abbreviations: see Mary.

Mariah

Origin/meaning: Hebrew 'bitter' or 'wished for child'.

A variation on Mary that has greatly increased in popularity, most likely because of the singer Mariah Carey.

Girls' Names

Mariana/Marianne
Origin/meaning: uncertain. Possibly Hebrew 'bitter' or 'longed for child'.
The Spanish and Italian diminutives of Mary (Maria), meaning 'little Mary'.
Variations and abbreviations: see Marion.

Marie
Origin/meaning: uncertain. Possibly Hebrew 'bitter' or 'longed for child'.
The French form of Mary.
Variations and abbreviations: see Mary.

Marietta
Origin/meaning: Hebrew 'bitter' or 'longed for child' plus Antoinetta (from the Roman Antonius family).
A contraction of Marie-Antoinette.

Marilyn
Origin/meaning: Hebrew 'bitter' plus Old English 'pool'.
A US combination of two popular names, Maria and Lyn. Its great popularity in the 1950s is undoubtedly due to the film star Marilyn Monroe (Norma Jean Baker), 1926–1962.

Marina
Origin/meaning: uncertain. Usually given as Latin 'of the sea'.
May also be a form of Mary q.v. Occasionally used in England in the Middle Ages.
Variation: Marinetta.

Marion
Origin/meaning: uncertain. Possibly Hebrew 'bitter' or 'wished for child'.
Marion means 'little Mary'. It has been used as an independent name since the Middle Ages, when Robin Hood and his Maid Marian are said to have flourished.
Variations: Marian, Mariana (It/Sp), Marianna (It), Marianne (Fr), Maureen (Ir). See also Mary.

Marjorie
Origin/meaning: Persian?/Greek/Latin 'pearl' or French/English 'daisy'.
This is a Scottish pet form of Margaret, used as an independent name since the 12th century. It has been a separate name for so long it has also become associated with the herb marjoram.
Variations: Margery, Marjory. See also Margaret.

Marlene (pron. Marrlayna)
Origin/meaning: Hebrew 'bitter' plus 'of Magdala'.
A combination of Maria and Lene (a common German short form of Magdalena). It was created for Marlene Dietrich the German singer/actress whose full name is Maria Magdalena von Losch.

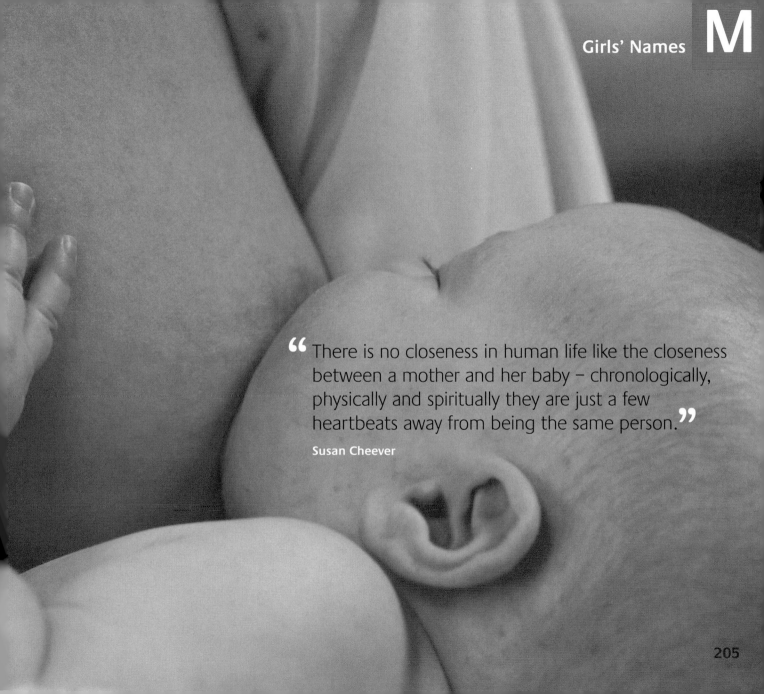

"There is no closeness in human life like the closeness between a mother and her baby – chronologically, physically and spiritually they are just a few heartbeats away from being the same person."

Susan Cheever

Girls' Names

Marsha
Origin/meaning: Latin 'of Mars' (the Roman god of war), i.e. 'warlike'.
An American form of Marcia q.v. which reflects the American pronunciation.

Martha
Origin/meaning: Aramaic 'lady'.
Martha was the sister of Mary Magdalen and Lazarus. She was upbraided by Christ for allowing her chores to distract her from sitting and listening to him. Martha is appropriately the patron saint of housewives.
Variations and abbreviations: Marja (Russ), Marta (It), Marte, Marthe (Fr), Mari, Martie, Martita, Marty.

Martina
Origin/meaning: Latin 'of Mars' (the Roman god of War) i.e. 'warlike'.
Variations and abbreviations: Marta, Martie, Martine (Fr), Marty, Martyna, Tina.

Mary
Origin/meaning: uncertain. Possibly Hebrew 'bitter' or 'wished for child'.
The name in Hebrew was spelt only with consonants – MRYM. The Latin form Maria was the intermediate source of Mary. The English form Mary developed from the French form Marie. Scotland, which at the time was more closely allied with France than England, tended to retain the original French form. In the 18th century, after a period in decline, the name began to come back into favor, often in the Latinized form Maria, so that by the 19th century it was again one of the commonest names in Britain. The Irish form Máire (similar to the Welsh Mair and Scottish Mora) has re-established itself since the beginning of the 20th century.
Variations and abbreviations: Maia, Maidie (Wel), Mair, Maire (Fr), Mairi (Scot), Maja (Ger), Mame, Mamie (US), Manette (Fr), Manon (Fr), Mara, Maria (It/Sp), Mariam, Mariamne, Marian, Mariana, Marianna, Marianne, Marice, Marie (Fr), Mariel, Marietta, Mariette (Fr), Marilyn, Marion, Mariquilla, Mariquita (Sp), Maris, Marisa, Mariska, Marita (Sp), Maritsa, Marja (Slav), Marla, Marya, Maryann, Maryanne, Marysa, Maryse, Marscha (Russ), Masha (Russ), Maura, Maure (Ir), Maureen (Ir), Maurita, May, Meriel, Meryl, Mimi, Minette, Minnie, Minny, Miriam, Mitzi, Moira (Scot), Moire (Scot), Mollie, Molly, Moyra (Scot).

Matilda
Origin/meaning: Old German 'battle strength'.
This is the Latin form of an Old German name, introduced into England by the Normans. Matilda was the name of William the Conqueror's wife.
Variations and abbreviations: Mahault (Med Fr), Maitilde (Ir), Majalda (It/Port), Matelda (It), Mathilda, Mathilde (Fr/Ger), Matilde (Sp), Mattie, Matty, Maud, Maude, Maudie, Mawt (Med Eng), Mechtilde, Tilda, Tillie, Tilly.

Maud
Origin/meaning: Old German 'battle strength'.
A medieval form of Matilda. Tennyson's poem 'Maud', 1855, may have contributed to its popularity in the 19th century.
Variations and abbreviations: Maude, Maudie, Mawt. See also Matilda.

Maureen
Origin/meaning: uncertain. Possibly Hebrew 'bitter' or 'wished for child'.
This is the Irish diminutive of Mary (Maire) and means 'little Mary'.

Mavis
Origin/meaning: French 'song thrush'.
A modern name which first appeared in the 19th century.
See also Merle.

Mawusi (pron. Mawusée)
Origin/meaning: Ewe 'in the hands of God'.
A name from Ghana.

Maxine
Origin/meaning: Latin 'little great one'.
A French feminine diminutive of Max, the short form of Maximilian q.v. It dates from the 19th century.

May
Origin/meaning: Sanskrit 'growth', 'burgeoning'. The name of the fifth month of the year.
In the 20th century this name has usually been given as the name of the month. May was considered a special month in the year, associated with festivity. In the 18th and 19th centuries May was often used as a familiar form of Mary or of Margaret.
Variations: Mae, Mai (Fr/Ger/Scand), Maye.

Meave
Origin/meaning: Old Irish 'joy'.
A name from Irish legend, Meave was considered the equivalent of the English Mab, the fairy who manipulated men's dreams.

Meena
Origin/meaning: Sanskrit, either from meen (fish) or meena (enamel work which shines like fishes' scales).

Meenakshi (pron. Meenakshée)
Origin/meaning: Sanskrit 'eyes like a fish'.
This is the equivalent of the English expression 'doe's eyes' and is a flattering description.

Meera (pron. Meeráh)
Origin/meaning: from the Rajasthan area, meaning obscure.
Meera was one of the most famous Hindu saints. She was a devotee of Krishna and wrote many poems about him. Gandhi gave this name to Jane, his adopted English daughter.

Girls' Names

Megan
Origin/meaning: Persian?/Greek/Latin 'pearl' or French/English 'daisy'.
This is a comparatively recent Welsh pet form of Margaret q.v. It seems to have been used first for Lady Megan Lloyd-George, 1902–1966, daughter of David Lloyd-George.

Melanie
Origin/meaning: Greek 'black', 'dark-haired'.
St Melania the younger, 383–439, was a rich woman who converted her husband to Christianity. Husband and wife then emancipated their slaves and gave away their wealth to the poor. The French version of the name was introduced in the 17th century by Huguenot refugees who fled to England.
Variations and abbreviations: Mel, Mela, Malania (It), Mélanie (Fr), Melinda, Melloney, Melly, Melony.

Melinda
Origin/meaning: uncertain. Sometimes given as 'loved' or 'dark-haired'.
This 20th-century name seems to be a combination of several names which are favorites in the US such as Melanie and Linda.
Variations and abbreviations: Linda, Lynda, Malinda, Melinde, Mindy (US)

Melissa
Origin/meaning: Greek 'bee' or 'Melissa officianalis' the Latin name for the herb lemon balm.
Used in pre-Christian Greece and by 16th and 17th-century poets to evoke that era. It is also much used in Italy probably because Ludovico Ariosto used the name in his epic poem 'Orlando Furioso', 1516. In the poem Melissa is a prophetess who lives in Merlin's cave and is able to change into different shapes.
Variations and abbreviations: Lisa, Lissa, Malissa, Mel, Melisa, Melitta, Milly, Missie, Missy.

Melody
Origin/meaning: Greek 'a song being sung'.

Mercedes
Origin/meaning: Spanish 'mercies'.
This is part of a standard Spanish description of the Virgin Mary, Maria de Mercedes – Mary of Mercies. The main word became a name in its own right.
See also Consuelo, Mercy.

Mercy
Origin/meaning: Medieval Latin 'pity'.
This name was one of the abstract virtue names popular with the 17th-century Puritans.
Variation: Merry.

Meredith
Origin/meaning: Welsh 'great?/lord'.
This was a Welsh masculine first name, with the accent on the second syllable. It became a last name but it is now having a new life as a first name, this time mainly for girls.
Variations and abbreviations: Bedo (Wel), Maredudd (Wel), Meredudd (Wel), Merry.

Meriel
Origin/meaning: Old Irish 'bright sea'.
An old form of Muriel q.v.

Merle
Origin/meaning: French 'blackbird'.
This is a French last name which may indicate an ancestor who was fond of whistling. It was a family name of Estelle O'Brien Merle Thompson who used it to create the stage name Merle Oberon.

Meryl
Origin/meaning: Hebrew 'bitter' and Latin 'famous in war'.
A familiar form of the common double name Mary Louise, brought to prominence by the US actress Meryl Streep.

Mhonum
Origin/meaning: Tiv 'mercy'.
This is a Nigerian name.

Mia
Origin/meaning: uncertain. Possibly Hebrew 'bitter' or 'wished for child'. Sometimes Italian 'mine'.
A European short form of Mary (Maria) made familiar by the US actress Mia Farrow.
Variations and abbreviations: see Mary.

Michelle (pron. M'shell)
Origin/meaning: Hebrew 'Who is like the Lord?'.
A French feminine form of Michael q.v. It became common in the 1960s after the success of the Beatles song 'Michelle'.
Variations and abbreviations: Michaela (It), Michela (It), Michèe (Fr), Micheline (Fr), Mick, Mickie, Micky.

Mildred
Origin/meaning: Old English 'mild strength'.
This was the name of a Saxon saint who died about 700. The daughter of King Merewald of Mercia she was an abbess renowned for her gentleness. Mildred survived the influx of new names at the Norman Conquest because of the saint's great following.
Variations and abbreviations: Meldred (Med Eng), Mil, Mildrid, Millie, Milly.

Girls' Names

Millicent

Origin/meaning: Old German 'work-strong'.

This is the usual modern form of a name which goes back to the time of the Emperor Charlemagne, 742–814. He named his daughter Melisendra which was a popular name of the period. When the name first came to England it was in the Medieval French form Melisant.

Variations and abbreviations: Lissa, Mel, Melicent, Mélisande (Fr), Melisenda (Sp), Melisendra, Mellicent, Mellisent, Mellie, Melly, Milicent, Milli, Millie, Millisent, Milly.

Mimi

Origin/meaning: uncertain. Possibly Hebrew 'bitter' or 'wished for child'.

A European familiar form of Mary and Miriam.

Minnie

Origin/meaning: Hebrew 'bitter' or Old German 'helmet of resolution'.

A Scottish familiar form of Mary q.v. now used as an independent name, or a short form of Wilhelmina, like the German Minna.

Variations and abbreviations: Min, Mina, Minna, Minne, Minni, Minka (Slav). See also Mary and Wilhelmina.

Mirabel

Origin/meaning: Latin 'wonderful'.

A name found occasionally since the Middle Ages.

Variations and abbreviations: Mira, Mirabella, Mirabelle (Fr).

Miranda

Origin/meaning: Latin 'admirable'.

This name was probably invented by Shakespeare who used it for the heroine of his play 'The Tempest', 1611.

Variations and abbreviations: Mira, Myra. See also Fiona, Lorna, Pamela, Perdita, Stella, Vanessa, Wendy.

Miriam

Origin/meaning: uncertain. Possibly Hebrew 'bitter' or 'wished for child'.

This is a translation of the name which appears in Hebrew as MRYM and is translated elsewhere as Mary. The two translations have come to be accepted as totally independent names. Miriam was the name of the sister of Moses.

Variations and abbreviations: Mariamne, Mimi, Mirjam (Ger), Miryam (Fr), Mitzi (US), Myrjam (Ger).

Miucca

Origin/meaning: unknown, but familiar in fashion circles for being the name of the iconic Italian fashion designer Miucca Prada.

Modron

Origin/meaning: a goddess of Welsh Celtic legend, mentioned in the collection of Welsh folk tales, 'The Mabinogion'.

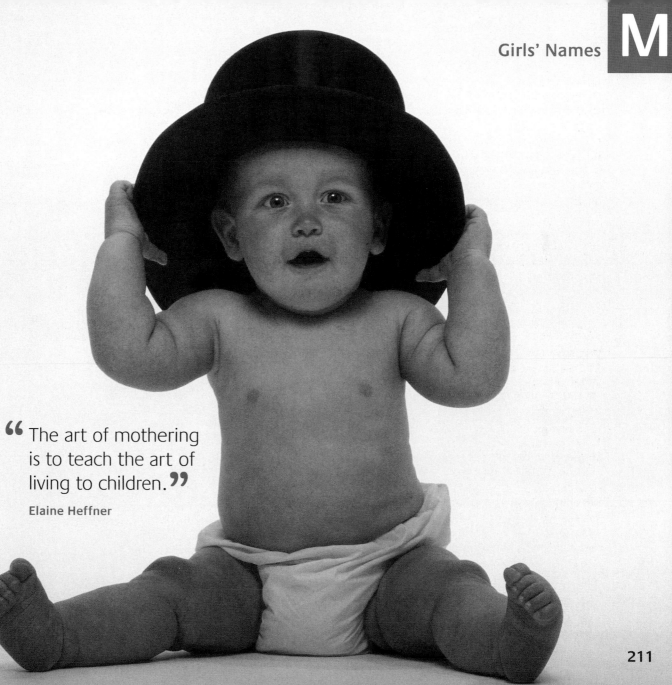

> **"** The art of mothering is to teach the art of living to children. **"**
>
> Elaine Heffner

Girls' Names

Mohini
Origin/meaning: Sanskrit 'bewitching woman'.
In some Hindu legends, the name taken by Vishnu when he took on the guise of a beautiful woman in order to interrupt the meditation of Shiva because it was feared the energy of such intense thought would destroy the universe.

Moira (pron Moy-ra)
Origin/meaning: uncertain. Possibly Hebrew 'bitter' or 'wished for child'.
This is a Scots version of Mary q.v. now used as an independent name.
Variation: Moyre. See also Mary.

Molly
Origin/meaning: uncertain. Possibly Hebrew 'bitter' or 'wished for child'.
A familiar form of Mary, often used as an independent name.
Variation: Mollie.

Mona
Origin/meaning: Old Irish 'little noble one'.
At the beginning of the 19th century it became more widespread as people became interested in native Irish language and culture.

Mona
Origin/meaning: Arabic 'hope'.
A Muslim name quite unconnected with the Irish name above.

Monica
Origin/meaning: uncertain. Sometimes given as Latin 'monk' or 'adviser'.
St Monica, 331–387, was the mother of St Augustine. In his writings he explains how she contributed to his conversion to Christianity.
Variations and abbreviations: Mona, Monika (Ger), Monique (Fr).

Morna
Origin/meaning: Gaelic 'affection'.
In James Macpherson's translation of the 3rd-century Ossianic poems published in the 18th century, Morna is the name of Fingal's mother.

Morowa
Origin/meaning: Akan 'queen'.
A Ghanian name. Other African names meaning 'queen' are Thema (also used in Ghana) and Torkwase (used in Nigeria).

Morwenna

Origin/meaning: Old Welsh 'wave', 'of the sea'.
St Morwenna was a 6th-century saint, the patron of Morwenstow in Cornwall, and the name was used in Cornwall as well as Wales.
Variations and abbreviations: Morwen, Morwinna, Mwynen.

Mukta (pron. Mookta)

Origin/meaning: Sanskrit 'pearl'.
A name found throughout India. It honors Muktabai, a saintly Hindu woman.

Muriel

Origin/meaning: Old Irish 'bright sea'.
This is the Norman version of a Celtic name.
Variations: Meriel, Miriel, Murial, Muriella, Murielle.

Muteteli (pron. Mutetáyli)

Origin/meaning: Rwanda 'dainty'.
A name used in the Central African Republic of Rwanda.

Myfanwy (pron. Mivvánwee)

Origin/meaning: Welsh 'my rare one'.
Variations and abbreviations: Fanny, Myfi, Myvanwy.

Myra

Origin/meaning: a coined literary name used in the 17th and 18th centuries. Myra was the name of a city in Asia Minor. It was used by, among others, Sir Fulke Greville (Lord Brooke), 1554–1628, who may have originated it, and George Crabbe, 1754–1832. It is also used as a short form of Miranda, Miriam and Muriel q.v.
Variations: Mira, Myrrah.

Myrtle

Origin/meaning: Greek. The name of a sweet-smelling flowering shrub.
There are several legends and superstitions surrounding the myrtle tree. These include the belief that eating myrtle leaves conferred the power to detect witches. The myrtle was also associated with Venus the Greek goddess of love.
Variations and abbreviations: Mertle, Mirtle, Myrrha, Myrta, Myrtah, Myrtice, Myrtilla.

N

Nadia (pron. Nahdeea)
Origin/meaning: Russian 'hope'.
This is the typical familiar form of the Russian name Nadezhda.
Variations and abbreviations: Nada, Nadina (It), Nadine (Fr), Nadja. See also Hope.

Nadika
Origin/meaning: Sanskrit 'river'.
A 'nadika' is also a measurement of time equaling 360 'pranas' (breaths) or 24 minutes.

Najma (pron. Naíma)
Origin/meaning: Arabic 'benevolent'.
A popular Muslim name.
Variation: Naeemah.

Nalini
Origin/meaning: Sanskrit 'lovely'.

Nancy
Origin/meaning: Hebrew 'graceful'.
A derivative of Hannah and Ann q.v.

Nanette
Origin/meaning: Hebrew 'graceful'.
A diminutive of Nan, a familiar form of Ann q.v. now found as an independent name. It enjoyed a short vogue in the wake of the musical 'No, No, Nanette'.

Naomi (pron. Nayóhmee)
Origin/meaning: Hebrew 'joy', 'delight'.
This name is the equivalent of the medieval name Pleasance. At about the time that Pleasance was becoming obsolete Naomi came into use.

Nasreen
Origin/meaning: Parsi 'wild rose'.

Natalia

Origin/meaning: Latin 'birth', i.e. Christmas day.
This is a name derived from the phrase 'natale domini' (birth of the Lord). It used to be given to girls born at the Christmas season and is an exact equivalent of Noël/Noëlle q.v.
Variations and abbreviations: Natalie (Fr), Natalina (It), Natalja, Natalya, Nathalia, Nathalie, Natasha (Russ), Natty, Nettie.

Natalie

Origin/meaning: Latin 'birth', i.e. Christmas day.
The French and German form of Natalia q.v. currently popular in English-speaking countries.
Variations and abbreviations: see Natalia.

Natasha

Origin/meaning: Latin 'birth', i.e. Christmas day.
The Russian diminutive of Natalia. It has been used since the 19th century in Britain when Russian novels were popular.
Abbreviation: Tasha.

Nellie

Origin/meaning: Greek 'bright' or 'light'.
A familiar form of Eleanor or Helen, both of which have the same meaning, and occasionally of Cornelia q.v.
Variations and abbreviations: Nell, Nelly.

Nerissa

Origin/meaning: Greek 'sea nymph'.
Nerissa was one of the Nereids who were the daughters of the sea god Nereus.

Nerys (pron. Néh-rees)

Origin/meaning: Welsh 'lord'.

Nessa

Origin/meaning: Greek 'pure', 'chaste'.
An English familiar form of Agnes q.v. similar to the Welsh version, Nesta.
Variation: Nessie.

Netta

Origin/meaning: this is a familiar form of names ending in -et (such as Janet and Annette).
Variations: Nettie, Netty, Nita (Sp).

Girls' Names

Nicola

Origin/meaning: Greek 'victory of the people'.
This is the Latinized feminine form of Nicholas q.v. It has recently become extremely popular in Britain.
Variations: Colette, Nichola, Nicole (Fr), Nicoletta (It), Nicolette (Fr), Nikol (Ger/Dut), Nikoline (Ger).

Nicole

Origin/meaning: Greek 'victory of the people'.
The French feminine form of Nicholas. It is used in many other countries and is particularly popular in Australia.
Variations and abbreviations: see Nicola.

Nigella

Origin/meaning: Old Irish 'champion'.
A rare feminine form of Nigel q.v. It is the Latin feminine form of the Latin Nigellus. By a happy coincidence, it is also the Latin name for the flower Love-in-the-Mist.

Nina

Origin/meaning: Hebrew 'graceful', or Spanish 'small girl'.
A Russian diminutive form of Ann, this name came into use in England along with other Russian names like Natasha and Nadine.

Nita

Origin/meaning: a Spanish diminutive of names like Juanita and Anita.
Now used as an independent name. The English equivalent is Netta q.v.

Noëlle

Origin/meaning: French 'Christmas'.
This is a modern French feminine form of Noël created on the pattern of a French adjective.
Variation: Noëlla. See also Natalia.

Nona

Origin/meaning: Latin 'ninth'.
A name given to a ninth child or girl when people had large families. It is occasionally used today without any consideration of its meaning but for its pleasant easy sound.

Nora

Origin/meaning: Latin 'honor' or 'beauty'.
An Irish short form of Honora which has been popular since the Middle Ages. It may also be used as a short form of Eleanor and Leonora.
Variations: Norah, Noreen.

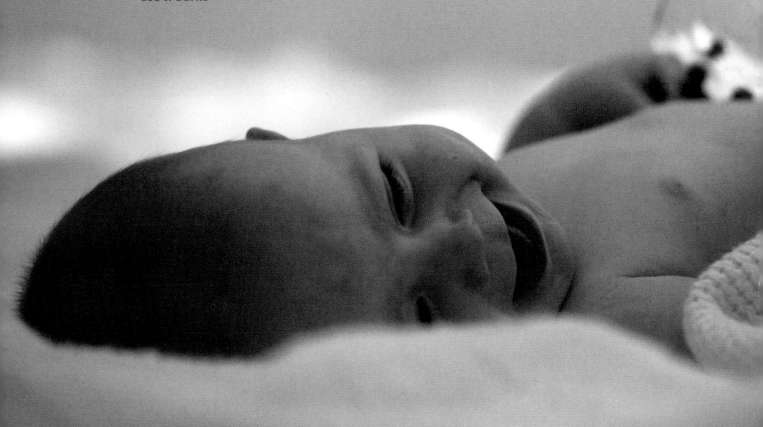

"People who say they sleep like
a baby usually don't have one."

Leo J. Burke

Girls' Names

Norma
Origin/meaning: Latin 'rule'.
This Latin word seems first to have been 'borrowed' as a name by Bellini for his opera 'Norma', 1831.

Nuala
Origin/meaning: Old Irish 'white shoulders'.
An Irish short form of Fenella through the form of Finnuala.

Nur Jehan
Origin/meaning: Sanskrit 'light of the world'.
This was the name of the wife of Jehangir q.v., 1569–1627, the third Mogul Emperor of India. Unlike Akbar q.v. his father, Jehangir was idle and pleasure-loving. Because of his weakness Nur Jehan was the effective controller of the Mogul empire. She is said to have relaxed by playing polo and shooting tigers. Nur Jehan is a popular Muslim name.
Variation: Nur Jahan.

Octavia
Origin/meaning: Latin 'eighth'.
A name given to an eighth girl or eighth child. Octavia, d.11 BC, was the sister of the Emperor Augustus and second wife of Mark Antony, who deserted her for Cleopatra.

Odette
Origin/meaning: Old German 'of the fatherland', 'rich'.
The German and French diminutive form of the Old German name Oda. One of the other variations is Odile and in the ballet 'Swan Lake', the black swan and the white swan, danced by the same dancer, have in effect the same name; one is Odile, the other Odette.
Variations and abbreviations: Oda, Odetta (It), Odile, Ottilie.

Olga
Origin/meaning: Old Norse 'holy'.
The root of this name is the Norse word helga – holy – and it is found in Russia because the founder of the Russian monarchy was a Viking.

Olive

Origin/meaning: Latin 'olive tree', 'olive branch'.

The olive, so vital to the southern European way of life, became a symbol of peace because in war the enemy would destroy the precious olive trees.

Variations and abbreviations: Liva, Livia, Livie, Livy, Nola, Nollie, Olivia, Olivette, Ollie, Olva.

Olivia

Origin/meaning: Latin 'olive tree'.

The Italian version of Olive q.v. It was popular during the 16th century when Shakespeare used it for the beautiful countess in 'Twelfth Night'.

Variations and abbreviations: see Olive.

Olwen

Origin/meaning: Old Welsh 'white footprint'.

In 'The Mabinogion', the collection of Welsh Celtic folk tales, Olwen was the daughter of a giant. Her beauty was so great that white trefoils appeared on the ground where she trod.

Variation: Olwyn.

Olympia

Origin/meaning: Greek 'from Olympia'.

Olympia was a religious centre in Ancient Greece and the site of the Olympic Games. The name is sometimes given as 'from Olympus', the mountain home of the gods and therefore 'celestial'.

Variations: Olimpe (Fr), Olimpia (It), Olympe (Fr), Olympias.

Ondine (pron. Ondeen)

Origin/meaning: Latin 'water sprite'.

The French form of Undine q.v.

Oni

Origin/meaning: Benin 'desired'.

A Nigerian name.

Oonagh (pron. Oohnah)

Origin/meaning: Old Irish, uncertain, possibly 'lamb'.

This name is also found in Scotland, another Celtic area.

Variations and abbreviations: Juno, Ona, Oona, Una.

Girls' Names

Opal
Origin/meaning: Sanskrit 'precious stone'.
This is one of the jewel names which have been used since the 19th century.

Ophelia
Origin/meaning: uncertain. Possibly Greek 'help' or 'serpent'.
This name seems to have been a literary name coined in the 16th century when classical Greek influence was strong. The best known example is Ophelia in Shakespeare's 'Hamlet', c.1600.

Oriana
Origin/meaning: Latin 'risen', 'dawn'.
A name coined in the 16th century as a flattering title for Queen Elizabeth I and the new era which she symbolized.

Oriel
Origin/meaning: uncertain, possibly Old German 'fire-strife' or Latin 'golden'.
This name was found in the Middle Ages and it probably has origins in a pre-Conquest name.

Orsola
Origin/meaning: Latin 'little she bear'.
An Italian variation of Ursula q.v.

Ottilie
Origin/meaning: Old German 'of the fatherland' or 'rich'.
One of the main variations, with Odile and Odette, of the Old German name Oda.
Variations and abbreviations: Otti, Ottilia (It), Ottoline.

P

Padma
Origin/meaning: Sanskrit 'lotus'.
A name found throughout Hindu texts for both men and women, although in modern times its use as a feminine name is more common.

Pamela (pron. Pámela or Paméela)
Origin/meaning: this name has no real meaning, although it is sometimes given as 'all-honey' because of a similarity to these Greek words.

This was an invention of Sir Philip Sidney's for his pastoral romance 'Arcadia', 1590. The great popularity of 'Arcadia' helped to establish Pamela as a name.

Variations and abbreviations: Pam, Pamella, Pammie, Pammy. See also Lorna, Miranda, Perdita, Ophelia, Vanessa, Wendy.

Parvati

Origin/meaning: Hindu 'mountain dweller'.
Parvati is a Hindu goddess, wife of Lord Shiva, one of the two major gods of modern Hinduism.

Parvin (pron. Parrvín)

Origin/meaning: Persian or Arabic. Meaning uncertain.
This Muslim name is found in both Pakistan and India.

Pascale

Origin/meaning: Hebrew/Latin 'of the Passover' or 'of Easter'.
A primarily French name, one of the most popular names in post-war France.
Variations: Pascaline (Fr), Pasqua (It).

Patience

Origin/meaning: Latin/Old French 'calm endurance'.
One of the abstract virtues used as names by 17th century Puritans in England and New England. In England it was sometimes used for men as well as women.
Abbreviation: Pat.

Patricia

Origin/meaning: Latin 'patrician', i.e. aristocratic.
The feminine form of Patrick q.v.
Variations and abbreviations: Paddie, Pat, Patrice (Fr), Patrizia (It), Patsy, Patti, Pattie, Patty, Tricia, Trish, Trisha.

Paula

Origin/meaning: Latin 'small'.
A German feminine version of Paul q.v. It has been used occasionally in England since the Middle Ages, probably to honor the Roman St Paula, 347–404.

Pauline

Origin/meaning: Latin 'small'.
A French feminine form of Paul q.v. and Paulinus often given to honor St Paulina.
Variations and abbreviations: Paola (It), Paolina (It), Paule (Fr), Paulene, Pauletta, Paulette (Fr), Paulina (Sp), Paulyn, Polly.

P

Girls' Names

Peggy
Origin/meaning: Persian?/Greek/Latin 'pearl' or French/English 'daisy'.
One of the English short forms of Margaret, probably the result of childish attempts to say Meggy.
Variations and abbreviations: Peg, Pegeen (Ir), Peggotty.

Penelope (pron. Pen-éll-opee)
Origin/meaning: uncertain. Possibly connected with the Greek word for a bobbin.
This is a name from Homer's poem 'The Odyssey'. Penelope was the wife of Odysseus. In Ireland it has sometimes been used to 'translate' the native Fionnghuala. It is used in English-speaking countries and, of course, Greece.
Variations and abbreviations: Pen, Penny, Poppy.

Perdita
Origin/meaning: Latin 'lost'.
This is a name made up by Shakespeare for his play 'A Winter's Tale'.

Perpetua
Origin/meaning: Latin 'continuous' or 'universal'.
The meaning of this name is similar to Constance. St Perpetua was martyred with St Felicity at Carthage in 203.

Peta
Origin/meaning: Greek 'stone'.
An occasional feminine form of Peter q.v.

Petra
Origin/meaning: Greek 'stone'.
This is the feminine form of Petrus, the Latin form given to the name Peter in medieval documents.
Variations and abbreviations: Peta, Piera, Petrina, Pierina. See also Petronella.

Petronella
Origin/meaning: Latin, from Petronius, a Roman family name.
In the Middle Ages this name was mistakenly believed to be the name of St Peter's daughter, a mythical St Petronilla who was honored as a saint.
Variations and abbreviations: Petronel, Petronia (It), Petronilla (It).

Petula
Origin/meaning: Latin 'pert' or 'seeker'.
A name made familiar by the English singer and actress Petula Clark.
Abbreviation: Pet.

" There are only two lasting bequests we can hope to give our children. One is roots; the other, wings. "

Hodding Carter, Jnr

Girls' Names

Philippa
Origin/meaning: Greek 'lover of horses'.
The Latin feminine form of Philip q.v.
Variations and abbreviations: Filippa (It), Filippina (It), Phil, Philipine, Pippa, Pippy.

Philomena
Origin/meaning: Greek 'love of song'.
St Philomena was the name of two early Roman martyrs. The renewed veneration of St Philomena in the 19th century brought about a revival of her name particularly in Italy.
Variations and abbreviations: Filippa (It), Filippina (It), Phil, Philomela (Ger), Philomene (Fr).

Phoebe (pron. Feebee)
Origin/meaning: Greek 'shining one'.
In Greek mythology Phoebe was another name for Artemis (Roman – Diana) the goddess of the moon. Her counterpart, Apollo, god of the sun, was also known as Phoebus. The usual Christian spelling was Phebe.
Variations: Febe (It), Phebe. See also Cynthia.

Phyllida
Origin/meaning: Greek 'leafy'.
A literary form of Phyllis q.v. much used in the 17th century.
Variations: Filada, Filide (It), Fillida, Philida, Phillada, Phillida.

Phyllis
Origin/meaning: Greek 'leafy'.
Phyllis was a Greek maiden who thought she had been forsaken by her lover and hanged herself. The gods pitied her and turned her into an almond tree. The name was used by Greek and Roman poets to signify an unspoiled country girl.
Variations and abbreviations: Fillis, Phillis, Phyl. See also Phyllida.

Pia (pron. Péeya)
Origin/meaning: Latin 'devout'.
This is an Italian and Spanish name occasionally used in English-speaking countries. The masculine, Pius, is almost never used, although it has been the name of twelve Popes.

Pippa
Origin/meaning: Greek 'lover of horses'.
An Italian short form of Philippa q.v. now used in Britain as an independent name.

Placida (pron. Plassida)
Origin/meaning: Latin 'calm'.
An adjective occasionally used as a girl's name.

Plaxy
Origin/meaning: Greek 'busy'.
An old Cornish name said to be a form of the Greek name Praxedes.

Polly
Origin/meaning: uncertain. Possibly Hebrew 'bitter' or 'wished for child'.
A familiar form of Mary, through Molly. Currently enjoying a minor vogue as an independent name.
Variations and abbreviations: see Mary.

Pollyanna
Origin/meaning: Hebrew 'bitter' plus Hebrew 'graceful'.
A double name equivalent of Mary-Anne (Polly is a familiar form of Mary).

Poppy
Origin/meaning: either a flower name or the Greek short form of Penelope.
Poppy has enjoyed a minor vogue in Britain in recent years.

Portia (pron. Pórsha)
Origin/meaning: either Latin 'sharing' or from Porcius, a Roman family name which may take its meaning from the word pig.
Variation: Porzia (It).

Primrose
Origin/meaning: Latin 'earliest rose'.
Flower names were a new fashion at the end of the 19th century. Primrose, being such a popular flower and associated with the beginning of spring, has always been one of the most frequently used.

Priscilla
Origin/meaning: Priscus was a Roman family name, probably meaning 'strict' or 'correct'.
This is a pre-Christian name adopted as a Christian name by 17th-century Puritans because it is found in the Bible.
Variations and abbreviations: Prisca (Ger/It), Priscille (Fr), Priska (Ger), Prissy, Cilla.

Priti (pron. Préetee)
Origin/meaning: Sanskrit 'love'.
Found throughout India. See Amanda, Amy.

Girls' Names

Prudence
Origin/meaning: Latin 'caution', 'discretion'.
A virtue name most common in the 17th century when it was popular amongst the Puritans. It is occasionally used in modern times.
Variation: Prue, Pru.

Prunella
Origin/meaning: Latin/French 'plum colored'.
This is a rare name.
Variation: Prunelle (Fr).

Q

Queenie
Origin/meaning: English 'little Queen'.
A late 19th-/early 20th-century girls' pet name, sometimes, at the height of its popularity, given as an independent name. It was originally given as a pet name for girls called Regina (the Latin word for Queen). In the 19th century girls named Victoria q.v. after the Queen, were also given Queenie as a nickname.
Variations and abbreviations: Queen, Queena, Queeny, Quenie. See also Victoria.

Querida
Origin/meaning: Spanish 'beloved'.

Quinta
Origin/meaning: Latin 'fifth', 'fifth born'.
The female equivalent of Quentin q.v. usually used either for a fifth daughter or a fifth child. Quintilla may also mean a girl born in July, the fifth month of the Roman calendar.
Variations: Quintilla (It), Quintina (It).

R

Rabia (pron. Rabéea)
Origin/meaning: Arabic 'spring'.
This is a popular Muslim name.
Variations: Rabiah, Rabiyyah.

Rachel

Origin/meaning: Hebrew 'ewe'.
Always a popular Jewish name this became a Christian name as well in the 17th century. At that time Rachael was the usual spelling and that old-fashioned spelling is again popular today.
Variations and abbreviations: Rae, Rachael, Rachele (It), Rachelle (Fr), Rahel (Ger), Rakel (Swed), Raquel (Sp), Raquela, Ray, Rey, Shelley, Shelly.

Radha

Origin/meaning: Sanskrit 'success'.
Found throughout Hindu texts but most famous for being the name of the favorite consort of Krishna. It is often used as a prefix to form other names.

Rajni (pron. Rjni)

Origin/meaning: Sanskrit 'night'.
Found throughout India.

Rajani

Origin/meaning: Sanskrit 'the night'.
In Hindu texts, a name of Durga, the wife of Shiva.

Ramona

Origin/meaning: Old German 'strength protection', 'counsel protection', i.e. 'strong', or 'wise protector'.
The Spanish feminine form of Raymond q.v. The best known feminine form, perhaps because of the song of the same name.
Variations: Raimonda (It), Raimunde (Ger), Raymonde (Fr), Reimunde (Ger).

Raphaela

Origin/meaning: Hebrew 'God has healed'.
A feminine form of Raphael q.v. used in Europe and occasionally found in English-speaking countries.
Variation: Raffaella (It).

Raquel

Origin/meaning: Hebrew 'ewe'.
Spanish form of Rachel q.v. given wider popularity because of Raquel Welch, the US film actress.

Rebecca

Origin/meaning: uncertain. Probably originates in a language of people neighboring Israel.
Sometimes given as 'faithful wife' or 'strongly bound'. It was an immensely popular name in the 17th century period of Biblical names, especially in Puritan New England.
Variations and abbreviations: Becca, Beckie, Becky, Bekki, Reba, Rebeca (Sp), Rebeka, Rebekah, Rebekka (Ger), Rivkah (Heb).

Girls' Names

Rehema
Origin/meaning: Swahili 'compassion'.
An East African name.

René
Origin/meaning: Greek 'peace'.
Short form of Irene q.v. sometimes given as an independent name.
Variation: Renie.

Rhoda
Origin/meaning: either Greek 'from Rhodes' (the isle of roses) or 'rose bush'.
This is one of the pre-Christian Greek names found in the Bible (Acts, ch.12) which was adopted as a Christian name by 17th-century Protestants. A quite separate Arabic name, Roda, means 'to be satisfied'.
Variations and abbreviations: Rhode, Rhody.

Rhona
Origin/meaning: uncertain. Possibly Old Welsh Rhonwen 'slender, fair' or Old German Ronalda 'power-might'.

Rhonda
Origin/meaning: uncertain. Possibly connected with the Rhondda area of Wales.

Rhonwen
Origin/meaning: Old Welsh 'slender, fair'.
A name sometimes considered to be the origin of the supposedly Saxon name Rowena.

Ria
Origin/meaning: either a short form of Maria meaning 'bitter' or a variation of the name of the goddess Rhea.

Rita
Origin/meaning: Persian?/Greek/Latin 'pearl' or Medieval French/English 'daisy'.
The short form of Margarita, the Spanish form of the name Margaret q.v.

Roberta
Origin/meaning: Old German 'fame bright'.
A feminine form of Robert q.v. found mainly in Scotland and also in Italy.
Variations and abbreviations: Bobbie, Roberte (Fr).

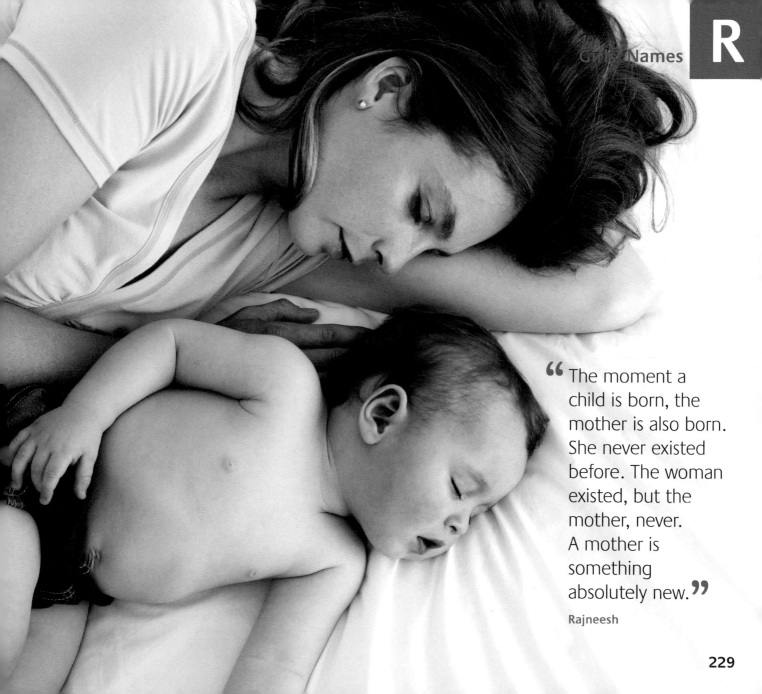

> **"** The moment a child is born, the mother is also born. She never existed before. The woman existed, but the mother, never. A mother is something absolutely new. **"**
>
> **Rajneesh**

R

Girls' Names

Robina
Origin/meaning: Old German 'fame bright'.
A feminine form of Robin q.v. found mainly in Scotland. In the US Robin is used for girls, although in Britain it is regarded as exclusively masculine.
Variations: Robbie, Robby, Robena, Robin, Robinia, Robyn.

Rokeya
Origin/meaning: Arabic 'she rises on high'.
This is a Muslim name.
Variation: Rukiya.

Roma
Origin/meaning: Italian, the city of Rome.
Occasionally used as a girl's name. A modern fashion.

Rona
Origin/meaning: uncertain. Possibly Old Welsh Rhonwen 'slender, fair' or Old German Ronalda 'power-might'.
The popularity of this name in Scotland suggests it is considered a feminine form of the Scottish masculine name Ronald and is a quite separate name from Rhona.

Rosalie
Origin/meaning: uncertain. Either Latin 'roses and lilies' or possibly Latin 'rosalia' a festival of flowers.
The original form Rosalia is still current in Italy but the name came to English-speaking countries via France and in the French form Rosalie.
Variations and abbreviations: Ros, Rosaleen (Ir), Rosalia (It), Rose, Rozalie, Roz.

Rosalind
Origin/meaning: Old German 'horse serpent'. Usually given as Spanish 'beautiful rose'.
The original Old German name was taken to Spain by the Goths. Despite the meaning the Old German is a flattering name since a serpent was considered a sacred creature (see Belinda). However in Spain it was naturally re-interpreted as the Spanish words 'rosa' – 'rose', and 'linda' – 'beautiful'.
Variations and abbreviations: Ros, Rosalinda (Sp), Rosaline, Rosalyne, Rosalynd, Roseline, Rosie, Roslindis, Rozalind.

Rosaline
Origin/meaning: Old German 'horse serpent'. Usually given as Spanish 'beautiful rose'.
A form of Rosalind q.v.
Variations and abbreviations: see Rosalind.

Rosamund

Origin/meaning: Old German 'horse protection', Latin 'pure rose'.
Like Rosalind q.v. this Old German name was re-interpreted in the Middle Ages, in this case using the Latin 'rosa' – 'rose', and 'munda' – 'pure'.
Variations and abbreviations: Ros, Rosamund, Rosamunda (Sp), Rosamunde (Ger), Rosemonde (Fr), Rosmunda (It), Roz, Rozamond, Rozamund.

Rosanna

Origin/meaning: a combination of the names Rose and Anna.
This name has been found in various spellings since the Middle Ages.
Variations and abbreviations: Roanna, Ronnie, Rosanne, Roseanna, Roseann, Rozanna, Rozanne, Zanna, Zanny.

Rose

Origin/meaning: Old German 'horse', Latin 'rose'.
This name was probably derived originally from the Old German Hros, meaning horse. The horse, like the serpent, was considered a god by the Saxons, as the white horses cut into chalk hillsides testify.
Variations and abbreviations: Ffion (Wel), Rhoda, Ross, Rosie, Rosy, Roze.

Rosemary

Origin/meaning: either a combination of two names Rose and Mary (Hebrew 'bitter') or a plant name.
The herb rosemary takes its name from the Latin words 'ros' – 'dew', and 'marinus' – 'of the sea'.
Variations and abbreviations: Mary Rose, Romy, Rosemarie (Fr), Rose Marie, Rosie, Rosy.

Rosita

Origin/meaning: Latin 'little rose'.
A Spanish diminutive of Rose q.v. Popular among Catholics as the pet name of St Rose of Lima, 1586–1617.

Roushan

Origin/meaning: Arabic 'dawn'.
A Muslim variation of Roxane q.v.
Variation: Roshanna.

Rowena

Origin/meaning: uncertain. Possibly Old English 'fame friend' or Old Welsh 'slender, fair'.
Variations and abbreviations: Rhonwen, Rona, Ronwen, Rhona.

Roxane (pron. Rocksahn)

Origin/meaning: Persian 'dawn'.
It was the name of the wife of Alexander the Great and has been used from time to time in literature.
Variations and abbreviations: Rossana (It), Roushan (Arabic), Roxana, Roxanna, Roxanne, Roxy. See also Aurora, Dawn, Zarah.

Girls' Names

Ruby
Origin/meaning: English 'red gemstone'.
A name taken directly from the name of a precious stone that became, along with other gemstone names, popular in 19th century England. While out of fashion for most of the 20th century, the start of the new century has seen the revival of such names.

Ruth
Origin/meaning: obscure. Sometimes given as Hebrew 'vision of beauty', also Medieval English 'compassion'.
Since Ruth was a Moabite it is unlikely this is a Hebrew name. A book of the Old Testament is given over to her story.
Variations: Ruthann, Ruthe, Ruthie.

S

Sabiah
Origin/meaning: Arabic 'morning'.
This is a popular Muslim name.
Variations: Sabah (East African), Sabera.

Sabina (pron. Sabeena)
Origin/meaning: Latin 'Sabine woman'. The Sabines were an ancient tribe whose lands bordered on Rome.
This Roman name survived because it was the name of several saints. In Britain Sabin became both a masculine and feminine variation in the Middle Ages. Sabina became the feminine form.
Variations: Sabin, Sabine (Ger/Fr), Sabyn, Savina (It), Savine (Fr).

Sabrina
Origin/meaning: the Latin name for the River Severn.
Milton in his play 'Comus' retells the Old British legend that Queen Guendolen, spurned by her husband Locrine, raised an army, defeated him and forced his mistress and his daughter Sabre to fly. In her panic Sabre jumped into the Severn but Nereus, a sea god, pitied her and changed her into a nymph. She became the goddess of the river which took its name from her.
Variation: Sabrin.

Sacha (pron Sah-shuh)
Origin/meaning: Ancient Greek 'defender of men'.
A short form of Alexander, or Alexandra q.v. frequently found recently as an independent first name for both boys and girls.
Variations and abbreviations: Sascha, Sasha.

Sadie

Origin/meaning: Hebrew 'princess'.
A familiar form of Sarah q.v.
Variations: Sadye, Saidee.

Sally

Origin/meaning: Hebrew 'princess'.
A form of Sarah q.v. which involves a typical change of letter from r to l. It has been given as a totally independent name.
Variations and abbreviations: Sal, Sallee, Sallie.

Salma

Origin/meaning: Arabic 'safe'.
A popular Muslim name that has become popular world-wide, and has recently become familiar thanks to the Hollywood actress Salma Hayek.
Variation: Solama.

Salome

Origin/meaning: Aramaic 'peace'.
This is a Greek form of the Hebrew word Shalom. It is the name given by tradition to the daughter of Herodias who danced before Herod in return for the head of John the Baptist. Despite this, it was a fairly popular Biblical name, given in honor of a follower of Jesus referred to in Mark's Gospel.
Variations: Saláma (Arabic), Salomé (Fr), Salomi, Salomy. See also Solomon.

Samantha

Origin/meaning: uncertain, possibly Aramaic 'listener' or feminine of Samuel ('name of God').
Samantha appears to be a mainly 20th-century name 'manufactured' by films and television. Particularly influential have been the characters of Tracy Samantha Lord played by Grace Kelly in the film 'High Society', 1956, and Samantha the young attractive witch in the widely distributed television series 'Bewitched', 1960.
Variations and abbreviations: Sam, Samanta (It), Samanthy, Sammie, Sammy. See also Darren, Tracey, Kelly.

Sandhya (pron. Sandayéah)

Origin/meaning: Sanskrit 'evening'.

Sandy

Origin/meaning: Greek 'defender of men'.
A familiar form of Alexandra q.v.
Variations: Sandi, Sandie.

S

Girls' Names

Sandra
Origin/meaning: Greek 'defender of men'.
The Italian short form of Alexandra (Alessandra) q.v.
Variations and abbreviations: Sandi, Sandie, Sondra, Zandra.

Sapphira (pron. Safféera)
Origin/meaning: Greek 'sapphire'.
This is a Biblical name which has been used occasionally since the Middle Ages.
Variations: Sapphire, Sephira.

Sarah
Origin/meaning: Hebrew 'princess'.
The Biblical Sarai was given to Abraham's wife by God. Although known in the Middle Ages, it only became widespread during the 17th century period of Biblical names. The spelling Sara is the Greek version.
Variations and abbreviations: Sadie, Sal, Sally, Sara, Saraid (Ir), Sari (Hung), Sarina, Sarita, Sarra, Sharai, Shari (Hung), Sorcha (Ir), Zara, Zarah, Zaria. See also Sharon, Soraya.

Saraid
Origin/meaning: Old Irish 'excellent' or Hebrew 'princess'.
Like Sorcha q.v. this native Irish name is also used as an equivalent of Sarah and therefore claims two meanings.

Sarswati (pron. Sarraswatti)
Origin/meaning: Hindu, the goddess of education, wife of Brahma.
A long-established name found throughout India. Sarswati is credited with the invention of Sanskrit. She is always portrayed as extremely beautiful.
See Athena.

Sati
Origin/meaning: Sanskrit 'virtuous wife'.
This was the name of the first incarnation of Parvati, wife of Shiva.

Scarlett
Origin/meaning: Middle English 'rich red'.
This word is assumed to have come from a Persian word for a rich cloth, usually deep red in color, called Saqirlat. Made famous by the heroine of Margaret Mitchell's book 'Gone With the Wind', 1936.
Variation: Scarlet.

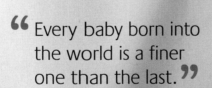

> **"** Every baby born into the world is a finer one than the last. **"**
>
> **Dickens (Nicholas Nickleby)**

Girls' Names

Selina
Origin/meaning: probably Latin 'heavenly'. Sometimes given as Greek 'moon'.
This comes from the French version, Céline. It first appeared as an English name at the end of the 17th century when French influence was very strong.
Variations and abbreviations: Celene, Celia, Celina, Céline, Selena, Selene, Selia, Seline. See also Celeste, Celia, Chandra.

Selma
Origin/meaning: Old German 'helmet of God'.
A short form of the rare Old English name Anselma.
Variation: Zelma.

Selma
Origin/meaning: Arabic 'secure'.
A popular Muslim name quite unrelated to the European name.

Senga
Origin/meaning: Greek 'pure', 'chaste'.
A Scottish name, thought to be simply a reversed spelling of Agnes.

Septima
Origin/meaning: Latin 'seventh'.
A name given to a seventh daughter or seventh child.

Seraphina
Origin/meaning: Hebrew 'burning', 'ardent'.
The name of one of the early saints.
Variations: Serafina (It), Seraphite (Sp).

Serena (pron. Seréena)
Origin/meaning: Latin 'calm', 'serene'.
A name found occasionally since the Middle Ages.

Shakira
Origin/meaning: Arabic 'be grateful'.
A Muslim name.
Variations: Shakila, Shakura (East African).

Shanti

Origin/meaning: Sanskrit 'tranquil'.
Originally a word used to denote the peaceful mental state achieved through meditation, in later Hindu texts Shanti appears as the name of the daughter of the deity Daksha.

Sharon

Origin/meaning: Hebrew place-name. Possibly also Hebrew 'princess'.
The phrase 'rose of Sharon' appears in the Song of Solomon. Rose-of-Sharon became abbreviated to simple Sharon.
Variations and abbreviations: Sharai, Shari, Sharron, Sharry, Sharyn.

Sheela

Origin/meaning: Sanskrit 'good character'.
Originally one of the six perfections to be striven for in Buddhism. It was not used as a female name until the late medieval period.
Variation: Sheila.

Sheila

Origin/meaning: Latin 'blind'. From the aristocratic Roman Caecilius family.
The Anglicized form of Shelagh/Sighile, which is itself the Irish form of Cecilia q.v.
Variations: Sheela, Sheelagh Sheelah, Sheilah, Shelagh Shelly.

Shelley

Origin/meaning: Old English 'clearing on a bank'.
A last name sometimes used as a feminine first name. Also a familiar form of names such as Michelle, Sheila, Shirley, Rachel, Rochelle.
Variation: Shelly.

Shena

Origin/meaning: Hebrew 'Jehovah has favored'.
Scots form of Joan or Jane, a phonetic spelling of the Scots Gaelic Sine.
Variations: Sheena, Sine.

Sherry

Origin/meaning: a familiar form of names like Chérie, Sharon, Charlotte, etc.
Sometimes given as an independent name.

Shirley

Origin/meaning: Old English 'bright clearing'.
An English place-name which became a last name. As a first name, it seems to be a direct result of Charlotte Brontë's novel 'Shirley', 1849.
Variations and abbreviations: Sher, Shir, Shirl, Shirlee, Shirleen, Shirlene, Shirline.

Girls' Names

Shobha
Origin/meaning: Hindu 'decoration', 'beauty'.
A name found throughout India.

Siân (pron. Shahn)
Origin/meaning: Hebrew 'Jehovah has favored'.
This is the native Welsh form of Jane q.v.
Variations: Siani, Sìne (Scot), Sinéad (Ir), Sioned, Siwan (Wel).

Sibyl
Origin/meaning: Greek. The name given to the women who put the prophecies of the oracles into words.
The name was introduced into England by the Norman Conquest. In the 19th century Disraeli's novel 'Sybil', 1845, revived interest in the name, although mistakenly spelt with the vowels reversed.
Variations and abbreviations: Cybil, Cybill, Sib, Sibelle, Sibbie, Sibby, Sibel, Sibilla (It), Sibylla, Sibylle (Fr/Ger), Sybil, Sybilla, Sybille.

Sidney
Origin/meaning: Latin/Greek 'follower of Dionysios'.
This aristocratic last name is a contraction of St Denis, a French place name. As a first name it had the additional boost to its popularity of being the last name of the much admired Elizabethan poet Sir Philip Sidney, 1554–1586.
Variations and abbreviations: Sid, Syd, Sydney.

Sidony (pron. Sidónee)
Origin/meaning: Greek/Latin 'fine cloth'.
The medieval word sendal, or sendon (from a Greek word) was used to describe a fine cloth and by implication in some cases, a winding sheet. Girls born on or about the date of the Feast of the Holy Sendon (winding sheet) were sometimes called Sidony.
Variations and abbreviations: Sid, Sidney, Sidonia (It), Sidonie (Fr/Ger), Sindonia, Zdenka (Slav).

Sienna
Origin/meaning: Latin 'from Siena'.
The name is taken from the Italian city and has become familiar as a first name because of Sienna Miller, the English actress.

Simone (pron. Séemon)
Origin/meaning: uncertain. Usually given as Hebrew 'hearkening'.
This is the French feminine form of Simon q.v.
Variations: Simona (It), Simonetta, Simonette, Simonne (Fr).

Sinead (pron. Shináyd)

Origin/meaning: Hebrew 'Jehovah has favored'.

This is the feminine form of Sean, the Irish form of John. It approximates to the English Jane.

Variations: Siàn (Wel), Sìne (Scot), Sinéidín (dim.). See also Joan.

Siobhán (pron. Shiváwn)

Origin/meaning: Hebrew 'Jehovah has favored'.

The Irish form of Joan q.v.

Sita

Origin/meaning: Hindu. Mythological. An incarnation of Lakohmi, the wife of Vishnu.

Sita was the wife of Rama, himself one of the incarnations of the god Vishnu. The adventures of Rama and Sita are told in many poems and stories including the famous epic poem 'The Ramayana'.

Sonia

Origin/meaning: Greek 'wisdom'.

This is a Slavic familiar form of Sophie q.v. It is particularly popular in Russia and is frequently found in Scandinavia.

Variations and abbreviations: Sonja, Sonnie, Sonya.

Sophia

Origin/meaning: Greek 'wisdom'.

The Italian form of Sophie q.v.

Variations and abbreviations: see Sophie.

Sophie

Origin/meaning: Greek 'wisdom'.

This is the English and French form of the name Sophia. The name came to England with the Hanoverians at the beginning of the 18th century. Sophie was the name of George I's daughter, and became fashionable very rapidly.

Variations: Sofia (Ger/It/Russ), Sofie, Sonia (Slav), Sonja, Sonya, Sophia (It), Sophy.

Soraya

Origin/meaning: Sanskrit/Persian 'good princess'.

An Arab name made more generally familiar by Queen Soraya, former wife of the late Shah of Persia.

Sorcha (pron. Sorshah)

Origin/meaning: Old Irish 'bright' or Hebrew 'princess'.

This native Irish name has come to be used as the Irish equivalent of Sarah and therefore has two meanings.

Girls' Names

Stacey
Origin/meaning: Greek 'resurrection'.
A short form of Anastasia q.v. which has become more popular than the original.
Variations and abbreviations: Stace, Stacy.

Stella
Origin/meaning: Latin 'star'.
This name was used from time to time in the Middle Ages to honor the Blessed Virgin Mary, one of whose titles is Stella Maris 'Star of the Sea'. Jonathan Swift, 1667–1745, gave the name Stella to a friend, Esther Johnson. It is a direct translation of Esther which is the Persian word for star.
Variations: Estella (It/Sp), Estelle (Old Fr), Estrella (Sp).

Stephanie
Origin/meaning: Greek 'wreathed', 'crowned'.
This is the feminine form of Stephen q.v. It was originally a French name, spelt Stéphanie.
Variations and abbreviations: Etiennette (Fr), Stef, Stefania (It), Stefanie (Ger), Steffie, Steph, Stephana, Stephani, Stephie, Stevana, Stevena.

Sudha (pron. Soo-thoh)
Origin/meaning: Hindu 'moon', 'nectar'.
See Chandra.

Sunita
Origin/meaning: Hindu 'well-behaved'
Found mainly in Central and Western India.

Sukey
Origin/meaning: Hebrew 'graceful white lily'.
Old-fashioned familiar form of Susan q.v. popular in the 18th century. Now becoming viable as an independent name.
Variation: Suki.

Susan
Origin/meaning: Hebrew 'graceful white lily'.
A short form of Susannah q.v. used in the 18th century and which by the 19th century had overtaken the original in popularity.
Variations and abbreviations: see Susannah.

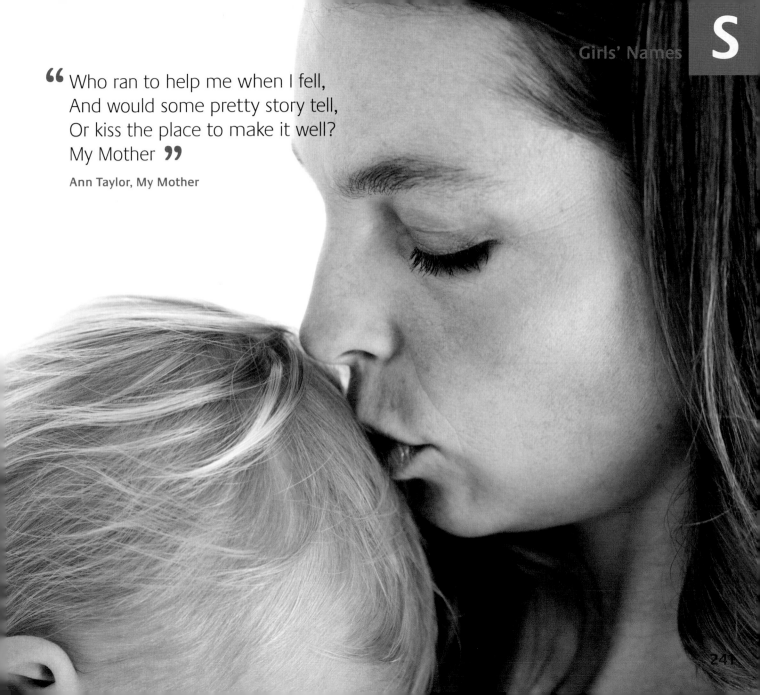

" Who ran to help me when I fell,
And would some pretty story tell,
Or kiss the place to make it well?
My Mother "

Ann Taylor, My Mother

Girls' Names

Susannah

Origin/meaning: Hebrew 'graceful white lily'.

This name, originally Shushannah, has the same meaning as Shushan, the royal city of Assyria. It is an ancient name yet was one of the most popular names of the mid-20th century. The (now apocryphal) story of Susannah and the Elders in the Old Testament made the name familiar in the Middle Ages and she was regarded as something of a heroine. Another Biblical Susanna is referred to in the New Testament.

Variations and abbreviations: Siusan (Scot), Sosanna (Ir), Sue, Sukey, Suki, Susana (Sp), Susanna (It), Susanne (Fr/Ger), Susette, Susi, Susie, Susy, Suzanna, Suzanne (Fr), Suzette (Fr), Suzi, Suzy, Zsa Zsa (Hung), Zusi.

Suzanne/Suzette/Suzan

Origin/meaning: Hebrew 'graceful white lily'.

French forms of Susannah q.v.

Sylvia

Origin/meaning: Latin 'of the woodland'.

This is the feminine alternative of Silvester (Silvius) q.v. The name spread to England from Italy mainly as a result of its use in Shakespeare's play 'The Two Gentlemen of Verona', c.1548, in which occurs the famous line 'Who is Sylvia, what is she?' From then it was used frequently in literature as a name for a fresh, young country maid.

Variations and abbreviations: Silva, Silvana (It), Silverie (It), Silvestra (It), Silvia, Silviana (It), Silvie, Sylviane (Fr), Sylvie (Fr), Sylvetta, Zilvia.

T

Tabitha

Origin/meaning: Aramaic 'antelope', 'gazelle'.

This is the translation of the Greek name Dorcas and both versions are given in the Acts of the Apostles.

Tacita (pron. Tássita)

Origin/meaning: Latin 'silent'.

Feminine of the Old Roman name Tacitus, still viable today, especially in Italy.

Tamara

Origin/meaning: Hebrew 'palm tree'.

A popular name in Eastern Europe but rare in English-speaking countries.

Variations and abbreviations: Tamar, Tammie, Tammy.

Tammy

Origin/meaning: Aramaic 'little twin'.
This is a pet form of the feminine versions of Thomas, Tamsin and Thomasina. It may occasionally be a short form of Tamara. It is now frequently given as an independent name.
Variations and abbreviations: Tam, Tammi, Tammie.

Tamsin

Origin/meaning: Aramaic 'twin'.
A feminine version of Thomas q.v. popular in Tudor times. It has continued to flourish in Cornwall and is currently enjoying a revival in popularity.
Variations and abbreviations: Tam, Tamasin, Tamasine, Tammy, Tamzin, Thomasin, Thomasina.

Tanya

Origin/meaning: uncertain. Possibly 'little queen'.
A Russian short form of Tatiana q.v. now used as an independent name.
Variations: Tanhya, Tania, Tonya.

Tatiana

Origin/meaning: uncertain, sometimes given as 'little father', 'little queen'.
One of the five most popular girls' names in Russia.
Variations and abbreviations: Tanhya, Tania, Tanya, Tonya.

Teri

Origin/meaning: Greek 'late summer'.
A short form of Theresa that has become a popular girl's first name. In recent times it has become familiar as a result of the actress Teri Hatcher.

Tess

Origin/meaning: uncertain, possibly Greek 'from Tharasia' or 'reaper'.
An English short form of Theresa q.v. now used as an independent name. May sometimes be given to a fourth child because of the Greek word tessara – four.
Variations: Tessa, Tessie, Tessy.

Thea

Origin/meaning: Greek 'goddess'.
This may be used as an independent name or as a short form of names beginning or ending with Thea such as Theadora.

Girls' Names

Thelma
Origin/meaning: literary, invented by Marie Corelli for her novel 'Thelma: a Norwegian Princess', 1887.

Theodora
Origin/meaning: Greek 'gift of God'.
The feminine form of Theodore q.v.
Variations and abbreviations: Dora, Fedora (Russ), Fjodora (Russ), Teodora (It), Thea, Theo.

Theresa
Origin/meaning: obscure, possibly Greek 'from Tharasia' or 'reaper'.
This name first took root in Spain. Its sudden introduction to the rest of Catholic Europe was due to the popularity of St Teresa of Avila, 1515–1582, the Spanish nun and mystic. In the 19th century the name received an additional boost to its popularity because of the French St Thérèse of Lisieux, 1873–1897. She was a nun who died of tuberculosis at the age of 24 but whose autobiography was widely read.
Variations and abbreviations: Teresa (Sp/It), Terese, Theresita (Sp), Teressa, Terri, Terrie, Terry, Tess, Tessa, Tessie, Tessy, Thérèse (Fr), Theresia (Ger), Tracey, Tracy.

Thora
Origin/meaning: Old Norse 'strength', 'thunder'.
This is a Scandinavian feminine name from Thor, the Norse god of war and thunder. Its use is comparatively recent in English-speaking countries.
Variations: Thorina, Thyra, Tora (Swed), Tyra.

Tiffany
Origin/meaning: Greek 'manifestation of God'.
Medieval English form of Theophania. In France Theophania was shortened to Tiphaine from which the English short form of Tiffany developed. In the 1990 US census it was in the top 3% as first name for females of all ages.

Tiger Lily
Origin/meaning: taken from the flower and familiar as a first name since being used as a name by British celebrity, the late Paula Yates, for her daughter with INXS star, Michael Hutchence, now also deceased.

Tilly
Origin/meaning: Old German 'battle strength'.
A pet form of Matilda.
Variations: Tillie.

Tina
Origin/meaning: a short form of names ending in -tine or -tina, e.g. Clementine, Christine.

Toni

Origin/meaning: Latin. From Antonius, one of the great Roman families.
This is a popular short form of Antonia q.v.
Variations: Tonia, Tonie.

Tracey

Origin/meaning: uncertain, possibly Greek 'from Tharasia' or 'reaper'.
This is an English familiar form of Theresa.
Variations: Tracie, Tracy.

Tricia

Origin/meaning: Latin 'patrician'.
A popular short form of Patricia, often used as an independent name.
Variations: Trish, Trisha.

Trudy

Origin/meaning: Old German 'strength' or 'spear strength'.
This is a short form of Gertrude which in the second half of the 20th century has been more popular than the original.
In Scandinavia and Germany it may refer back to Thrudhr, one of Thor's daughters, who was one of the twelve Valkyries.
Variations: Druda, Traude (Ger), Traute (Ger), Trude (Den), Trudel, Trudi, Trudie.

U

Ulla

Origin/meaning: Latin 'little she bear' or Old German/Old English 'wolf ruler'.
A short form of either Ursula or Ulrike used as an independent name. It is most popular in Scandinavia. The Scandinavian influence brought the name to Scotland.

Ulrike

Origin/meaning: Old German/Old English 'wolf ruler'.
The feminine of Ulrich.
Variations and abbreviations: Ulla, Ulrica (It), Ulricha, Ulrika (Scand).

Uma

Origin/meaning: Hindu. A goddess, one of the incarnations of Parvati, wife of the great god Shiva.

U

Girls' Names

Una (pron. Yéwna)
Origin/meaning: Latin 'one'.
A name first used by Spenser in his poem 'The Faeri Queen'. Sometimes, pronounced Oona, it is also used as a variant spelling of the Irish Gaelic name Oonagh.

Undine
Origin/meaning: Latin 'water sprite'.
A name invented by the 16th-century Swiss alchemist and astrologer Paracelsus from the Latin word unda, meaning wave. He used it to describe a water sprite.
Variation: Ondine (Fr).

Ursula
Origin/meaning: Latin 'little she-bear'.
St Ursula (probably 3rd or 4th century) was one of the martyrs of the Roman Empire. She and her companions were martyred for their Christianity by the Huns at Cologne. The discovery of a vast cache of bones at Cologne in the 12th century was used to support the story.
Variations and abbreviations: Orsa, Orsola (It), Ulla, Ursa, Ursala, Ursel, Ursina (It), Ursola (Sp), Ursule (Fr), Ursulina, Uschi (Ger). See also Orson.

Usha (pron. Oosha)
Origin/meaning: Sanskrit 'dawn'.
Found throughout Hindu texts including as the daughter of heaven, renowned for her beauty.

V

Valentina
Origin/meaning: Latin 'strong', 'healthy'.
The feminine version of Valentine q.v. although occasionally girls are also called by the original version.
Variations and abbreviations: Val, Valentine.

Valerie
Origin/meaning: Latin 'strong', 'influential'. From the patrician Roman family of Valerius.
The English feminine form of this name was brought over from France in the 19th century as Valérie.
Variations and abbreviations: Val, Valeria (It), Valeriane, Valérie (Fr), Valery, Valerye, Valeska (Slav).

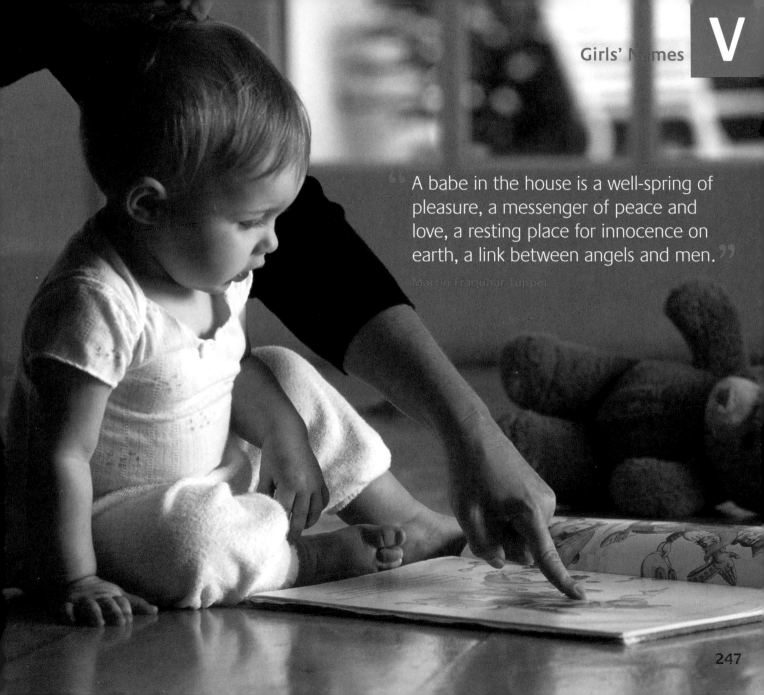

"A babe in the house is a well-spring of pleasure, a messenger of peace and love, a resting place for innocence on earth, a link between angels and men."

Martin Farquhar Tupper

Girls' Names

Vanessa
Origin/meaning: a pet name invented by the 18th-century writer Jonathan Swift for his friend Esther Vanhomrigh. He amalgamated the first syllable of her last name with -essa, a short form of Esther.
Variations and abbreviations: Nessa, Vanna.

Varsha
Origin/meaning: Sanskrit 'rain'.
A name found throughout India.

Veena
Origin/meaning: Sanskrit 'sitar'.
A name found throughout India. In Indian mythology this instrument is used by Narad (pron. Nard) the messenger of the gods.

Velma
Origin/meaning: Old German 'helmet of resolution'.
A short form, popular in the US, of Wilhelmina q.v. from the German pronunciation.

Venetia
Origin/meaning: used since the Middle Ages and taken from Venice, the romantic city of northern Italy.

Vera
Origin/meaning: Latin 'true', Russian 'faith'.
Probably in England a 19th-century short form of Veronica q.v. now used as an independent name. It may however be a direct use of the popular Russian name which is pronounced Vyera, and which was used by several 19th-century lady novelists such as Ouida ('Moths', 1860).
Variations: Véra (It), Vere, Veria, Verla.

Verena
Origin/meaning: Old German 'defender', 'protector'.
A martyr whose feast falls on September 1st. The name's introduction to England was probably through Mrs Yonge's popular novel 'The Heir of Redclyffe'. Sometimes used as a short form of Veronica.
Variations and abbreviations: Rena, Véran (Fr), Verina, Verine, Verna.

Verity
Origin/meaning: Middle English word 'truth'.
Used since the 17th century when Puritans chose virtues and Biblical names as an alternative to Catholic saints' names.
Variation: Verily.

Veronica

Origin/meaning: Latin 'true icon/image'.
The name traditionally given to the woman who wiped the face of Christ with a cloth while he was walking to Calvary. The image of Christ's face was said to be left on the cloth she used. Not surprisingly perhaps she is patron saint of photographers.
Variations and abbreviations: Nicky, Ronnie, Vera, Verena, Veronika (Ger), Véronique (Fr), Vroni.

Vesta

Origin/meaning: the name of the Latin goddess of the hearth.
Occasionally found as a first name.

Vicky

Origin/meaning: Latin 'victory'.
Short form of Victoria q.v. now found as an independent name.
Variations: Vicki, Vickie, Vikki, Vikky.

Victoria

Origin/meaning: Latin 'victory'.
Rare in England before the reign of Queen Victoria, 1837–1901. Victoria was the Queen's second name and had been one of the names of her German mother, the Duchess of Kent.
Variations and abbreviations: Queenie, Vic, Vicki, Vickie, Vicky, Victoire (Fr), Victorine, Viktoria (Ger), Viktorine, Vita, Vitoria (Sp), Vittoria (It), Vittorina (It).

Vida

Origin/meaning: Hebrew 'beloved'.
A short form of feminine versions of David q.v., e.g. Davida.

Villette

Origin/meaning: Old German 'helmet of resolution'.
Regional French version of William q.v.
See also Wilhelmina.

Viola

Origin/meaning: Latin 'violet flower'.
This Latin word for a violet was used occasionally during the Middle Ages as a feminine first name. It was chosen by Shakespeare for his heroine in 'Twelfth Night'.
Variations and abbreviations: Vi, Violante, Viole, Vye. See also Yolande, Violet.

Girls' Names

Violet

Origin/meaning: Latin 'the violet flower'.

The English word violet is first found as a name in Scotland in the 16th century, but it was not until the 19th century that the name became fashionable in England, along with many other flower names. In the language of flowers, Violet was given as a name which implied innocence and love of truth.

Variations and abbreviations: Vi, Violante (Fr), Violetta (It), Violette (Fr), Vye. See also Ianthe, Yolande, Viola.

Virginia

Origin/meaning: either Latin from the Patrician Roman family Verginius (spring) or Latin 'maidenly', 'virginal'.

The American plantation (later State) of Virginia, was named by Sir Walter Raleigh to honor Elizabeth I, England's Virgin Queen in 1584.

Variations and abbreviations: Ginger, Ginni, Ginnie, Ginny, Jinny, Jinney, Verginia, Virgie, Virginie (Fr).

Vita

Origin/meaning: Latin 'life', 'full of life'.

This Latin word was not used as a name until comparatively recently. Sometimes it is a short form of similar names, e.g. Victoria.

Vivian

Origin/meaning: Latin 'full of life'.

In the 19th century Tennyson used Vivien, which is based on the French form Vivienne, for one of his poems of the Arthurian legends, 'Vivien and Merlin' and the poem helped to popularize the name.

Variations and abbreviations: Bibiana, Viv, Vivien, Viviana (It), Viviane (Ger), Vivianne, Vivie, Vivienne (Fr), Vivyan. See also Vita.

Voletta

Origin/meaning: Old French 'a veil'.

Variations and abbreviations: Volet, Vollet (both pron. Vollay).

W

Wallis

Origin/meaning: Old Scots 'from Wales', 'foreign'.

A last name used as a girl's first name – a common practice in the Southern United States. Established more generally because of the US-born Mrs Wallis Simpson who married Edward VIII in 1937 and became the Duchess of Windsor.

Wanda

Origin/meaning: uncertain. Possibly Old German 'stem' or 'branch'. Sometimes given as 'wanderer'.
Very popular in Germany at the end of the 19th century, it was introduced into England by the novelist Ouida, who gave the name to the heroine of her book 'Wanda', 1883.
Variations: Vanda (It), Wenda.

Wendy

Origin/meaning: invented by J. M. Barrie for his book 'Peter Pan', 1904.
Apparently he had the idea because Margaret Henley, the small daughter of a friend, nicknamed him 'friendy-wendy'.
Variations: Wendi, Wendie, Wendye. See also Fiona, Lorna, Miranda, Ophelia, Pamela, Perdita, Vanessa.

Wilhelmina

Origin/meaning: Old German 'will helmet' i.e. 'helmet of resolution'.
A feminine form of William q.v. brought to England from the Netherlands and Germany during the 18th century partly because of the influence of the Dutch and Hanoverian members of the Royal family.
Variations and abbreviations: Billie, Billy, Guglielma (It), Guillema, Guillemette (Fr), Guillelmina (Sp), Guillelmine (Fr), Gullelma, Min, Mina, Minna, Minni, Minnie, Minny, Valma, Velma, Vilhelmina (Slav), Villette (Fr), Vilma, Wilella, Wilhelmine, Willa, Willamina, Williamina, Wilma, Wilmette, Wylma.

Willa

Origin/meaning: Old German 'helmet of resolution'.
Short form, popular in the US, of Wilhelmina.

Winifred

Origin/meaning: Old German 'peaceful friend', Old Welsh 'blessed reconciliation'.
Although this name is traditionally given the first meaning it is equally likely that it is the English version of the Old Welsh name Gwenfrewi (through the Latin Wenefreda), which means 'blessed reconciliation'. Winifred became popular in England in the 16th century but has been replaced in popularity by the shortened version, Freda.
Variations and abbreviations: Freda, Fredi, Freddie, Venefrida (It), Wenefrede, Wenefride, Winefred, Win, Winnie, Winnifred, Winny, Wyn.

Winona

Origin/meaning: Sioux Indian 'first born daughter'.
Variation: Wenona.

X

Xanthe (pron. Zanthee)
Origin/meaning: Greek 'yellow'.
Variation: Xantha.

Xenia (pron. Zennia)
Origin/meaning: Greek 'hospitable', 'guest'.
Variations and abbreviations: Xena, Zena, Zenia.

Y

Yasmin
Origin/meaning: Arabic/Persian 'jasmine flower'.
The Arab original of the better known English form Jasmine q.v.
Variation: Yamina. See also Jasmine.

Ynez
Origin/meaning: Greek 'pure', 'chase'.
A spelling of Inez, the Spanish form of Agnes q.v.

Yolande
Origin/meaning: Latin 'violet flower'.
A French name which developed from Violaine, or Violante, Medieval French forms of Viola, the Latin word for violet.
Variations and abbreviations: Iola, Iolande (It), Iolanthe (Ger), Jolanda (It), Jolanthe (Ger), Yolanda (Sp), Yolanthe. See also Violet, Ianthe.

Yvette
Origin/meaning: Old German 'yew'.
Like Yvonne, a feminine version of Yves, the French form of Ivo.
Variations: Evette, Ivette.

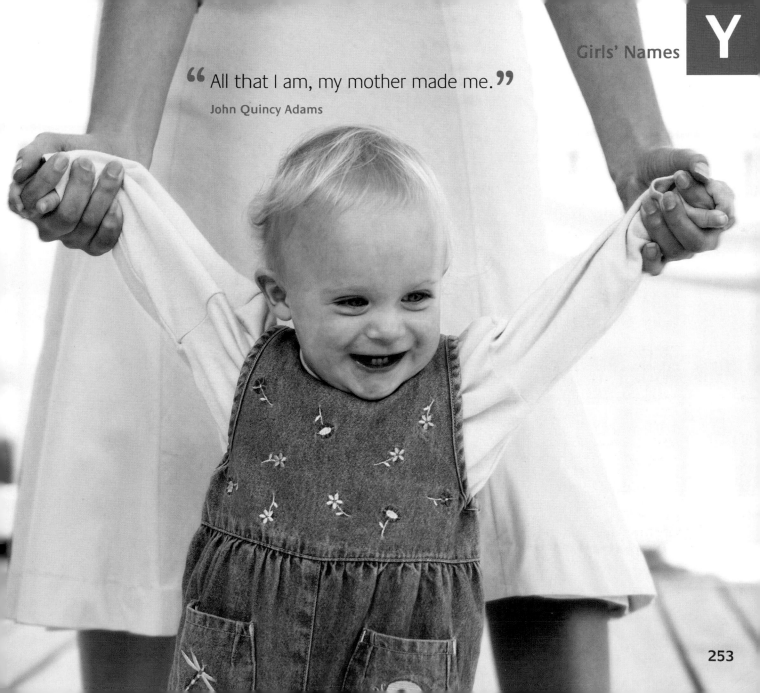

" All that I am, my mother made me. "

John Quincy Adams

Girls' Names

Yvonne
Origin/meaning: Old German 'yew'.
A French feminine version of Yves, Yvon, the French forms of Ivo.

Z

Zaha
Origin/meaning: origin unknown but familiar in architecture circles for being the name of the award-winning architect Zaha Hadid.

Zainab
Origin/meaning: Arabic 'beautiful'.
A Muslim name, Zainab was the eldest daughter of Mohammed.
Variation: Zainabu (E African).

Zakiya
Origin/meaning: Arab 'intelligent'.
This is a popular Muslim name.

Zandra
Origin/meaning: Greek 'defender of men'.
An abbreviation of Alexandra q.v.

Zarah
Origin/meaning: possibly Arabic 'flower', or Hebrew 'sunrise', 'dawn'. Possibly also a variant of Sarah 'princess'.
Variations: Zara, Zariah, Zerah, Zora. See also Dawn, Roxane.

Zarina
Origin/meaning: African 'golden'.

Zelda
Origin/meaning: uncertain. May be a contraction of Griselda, 'gray battle maid'.
A 20th-century name.

Zelma
Origin/meaning: Old German 'helmet of God'.
A form of Anselma/Selma q.v.

Zena
Origin/meaning: Greek 'hospitable'.
An Anglicized version of Xenia q.v.

Zillah
Origin/meaning: uncertain. May be Hebrew 'shade'.
A Biblical name (Genesis ch.4), one of the two wives of Lamech (the other one was Adah). Sometimes said to be a popular name among gypsies, it is otherwise rare. Antonia White used the name for the maid in her novel 'Frost in May'. It is also given to the maid in Emily Brontë's 'Wuthering Heights'.

Zinnia
Origin/meaning: a tropical plant.
One of the flower names occasionally used.

Zita
Origin/meaning: Etruscan 'young girl'. Sometimes given as Greek Zeta, the sixth letter of the Greek alphabet. It may sometimes be a short form of names, e.g. Rosita, which end in Sita or Zita.

Zoë
Origin/meaning: Greek 'life'.
Initially used because of its meaning to translate the Biblical Hebrew word for Eve, the mother of mankind, into Greek, Zoë became a name in its own right.
Variations: Zoa, Zoé (Fr).

Zoila
Origin/meaning: Spanish 'be cheerful'.
A rare but stylish name that was once popular in Spain and parts of Latin America. The male form is Zoilo.

Zsa Zsa (pron. Jhah-Jhah)
Origin/meaning: Hebrew 'lily' or 'princess'.
Hungarian form of Susan or Sarah made familiar by American/Hungarian actress Zsa Zsa (Sari) Gabor.

Zuleika (pron. Zoolíka)
Origin/meaning: Arabic 'fair', 'beautiful'.
A favorite Persian name. Max Beerbohm's satirical novel 'Zuleika Dobson', 1911, gave it some popularity in England.
Variation: Suleika (Ger).

" Where did you come from baby dear?
Out of the Everywhere into the here.... "

George MacDonald, At the back of the North Wind